# PREVENTING PHYSICIAN BURNOUT

# PREVENTING PHYSICIAN BURNOUT

## CURING THE CHAOS AND RETURNING JOY TO THE PRACTICE OF MEDICINE

**Paul DeChant MD,MBA**
**Diane W. Shannon MD,MPH**

*A Handbook for Physicians and Health Care Leaders*

ISBN-13: 9781539142959
ISBN-10: 1539142957
Library of Congress Control Number: 2016916463
CreateSpace Independent Publishing Platform
North Charleston, South Carolina

# *Praise for Preventing Physician Burnout*

DeChant and Shannon have addressed one of the central issues of health care today: physician burnout. It is hard to see how we can create the health care system we want and need on the backs of joyless and unengaged doctors. This well-written, practical book offers the prescription we need to address this crisis.

> Robert Wachter, MD
> Professor and Chair, Department of Medicine, University of California, San Francisco, and author of *The Digital Doctor: Hope, Hype, and Harm at the Dawn of Medicine's Computer Age*

DeChant and Shannon make a powerful and compelling argument for how to reduce physician burnout. The comprehensive case studies and physician interviews in this book clarify the symptoms, causes, and treatment for burnout. A must-read for health care leaders.

> John Toussaint, MD
> Chief Executive Officer
> ThedaCare Center for Healthcare Value

Dr. Paul DeChant and Dr. Diane Shannon provide extraordinary insights on a rarely discussed problem that undermines the very fabric of our health care delivery system: physician burnout. Drawing on research, case studies, and their own personal experience as physicians, they define the nature and extent of the problem and propose actions to mitigate this serious issue. This is a must-read for health care leaders and policy experts and in fact anyone trying to improve health care delivery.

> Joan Wellman
> Executive Vice President
> Simpler Healthcare
> Founder
> JWA Consulting

We live in a VUCA world that is increasingly volatile, uncertain, complex, and ambiguous. For many their joy and professional satisfaction has evaporated, as they feel more and more overwhelmed, isolated, and powerless in the chaos of organizational stress. I love the message of this book. It looks into the abyss of burnout and the distressed organization and asserts that there is hope for all of us to have joy return to our chosen professions from the C suite to the front line, if only we can embrace the principles of "Lean Done Right" and together build a better future on its core principles of respect and continuous improvement.

> Gene Lindsey, MD
> Former President and Chief Executive
> Officer
> Atrius Health

In this book, the authors are addressing one of the most critical issues in health care delivery today, and more importantly, doing so in a way that addresses the real challenges and opportunities to create the kind of health care systems that treat our patients well but also support our caregivers to serve the critical role that they play without having to damage themselves in the process.

> James Hereford
> Chief Operating Officer
> Stanford University Medical Center

Can physicians restore satisfaction and sustainability to the practice of medicine? Drs. Paul DeChant and Diane Shannon provide an inspiring vision of workplaces where health care teams can thrive and do their best work for the patients and families they serve.

> John E. Billi, MD
> Associate Vice President for Medical
> Affairs
> The University of Michigan

One of the most practical books that I have read regarding physician and overall health care system efficiency. The interviews and quotes from current industry leaders are invaluable. *Preventing Physician Burnout* not only provides real-world accounts of the many EHR reasons for the burnout epidemic, it also lays out clear and concise ways for health care leaders to address them.

> David K. Butler, MD
> Vice President for Information Services,
> EHR Optimization, and Transformation
> Initiatives
> Sutter Health

This is the book we've all been waiting for. A comprehensive, thoughtful discussion of the organizational causes and solutions to physician burnout. Any physician or health care leader will benefit from reading this book. Buy it today!

> Wayne M. Sotile, PhD
> Founder of the Center for Physician
> Resilience and Author of *The Resilient
> Physician: Effective Emotional Management
> for Doctors and Their Medical Organizations*

*Curing the Chaos and Returning Joy to the Practice of Medicine* does a fantastic job of assessing and diagnosing the underlying etiology of physician burnout. It also offers a prescription for the cure. Lean can't save the world, but it can save US health care.

> Montgomery Elmer, MD
> Family Physician
> ThedaCare

Using anecdotes as well as peer-reviewed research on the topic, Paul DeChant and Diane Shannon have created a handbook for physicians and health care leaders to learn from, with the hope that tangible steps will be taken to reduce or eliminate physician burnout. This is a book full of grit and resiliency as we all advocate for change in a system that often marginalizes doctors. Bravo!

Michelle Mudge-Riley, DO, MHA
Career Coach for Physicians

In this book, DeChant and Shannon focus attention on a critically important issue: the prevention of physician burnout. Addressing this problem and bringing joy back to the workplace will not only improve the lives of clinicians—it will improve the patient experience as well.

Paul Melinkovich, MD
President
Colorado Medical Services Board
Director of Community Health Services
Denver Health

*Curing the Chaos and Returning Joy to the Practice of Medicine* is essential reading. It delves into root causes and offers practical solutions for a critical problem that directly or indirectly affects all of us. Physician burnout has a domino effect on society, and solutions are available. If we continue to turn a blind eye to this problem, we are violating our Hippocratic Oath of "Do no harm" to our colleagues and the many who depend on them.

Monica Broome, MD
Assistant Professor
University of Miami Miller School of
Medicine
Master Trainer
Institute for Healthcare Communication

When we are ill and vulnerable, what we most need is compassionate and expert care. Yet if our caregivers are themselves stressed beyond their limits, that care will inevitably suffer. This book highlights why this is an issue of pressing concern and illuminates the underlying causes of physician burnout. Most importantly of all, it points to a solution: the building of deep and respectful partnerships that engage all staff, and particularly doctors, in finding a better way of doing things. Better for patients, and better for the caregivers too.

David Fillingham
Former Chief Executive
Royal Bolton Hospital, United Kingdom

The phenomenon of physician burnout threatens the sustainability of our nation's health care system. Drs. DeChant and Shannon effectively tackle this complex problem and provide both physicians and health care leaders with a way to understand the multilayered contributors to the problem while providing concrete, operational interventions that can be implemented immediately. This handbook will ameliorate the paralysis many health care leaders feel when facing the crisis of burnout in their organizations.

Karen Weiner, MD, MMM
Chief Medical Officer
Oregon Medical Group

DeChant and Shannon provide a no-nonsense, plain-language explanation for the root causes of the international challenge of physician burnout and recommend practical steps to reduce burnout's drivers. They envision a clear path to burnout prevention that aligns so well with the medical home movement.

Paul Grundy, MD, MPH
Global Director of Healthcare
Transformation
IBM

Physician burnout is a dominant, heartrending reality of the health care industry, but this book offers a hopeful and practical way forward. You'll find renewed vision and an achievable pathway toward a working environment in which health care workers can truly thrive.

Peter Anderson, MD
President
Team Care Medicine

Though wellness programs and psychosocial support are important to ameliorate physician burnout, DeChant and Shannon go deeper by addressing root causes; the dysfunctional workplace, the changing health care landscape and a lack of physician empowerment and engagement to influence said workplace. The authors offer the Lean management system as a way to engage physicians to partner with health care leadership in order to rectify the chaotic, reactive, non-standardized, and inefficient state of the daily health care delivery system. *Preventing Physician Burnout* is a must read for those physicians and health care leaders who want to disrupt the status quo and lead change.

Craig T. Albanese, MD, MBA Senior Vice President, Chief Operating Officer New York-Presbyterian/Morgan Stanley Children's Hospital and Author of *Advanced Lean In Healthcare*

# CONTENTS

# Acknowledgments

We would like to thank the leadership of Simpler Healthcare for supporting our year-long effort to research and write *Preventing Physician Burnout.*

We are indebted to the clinicians, researchers, and Lean practitioners who dedicated their time to enriching our understanding of physician burnout. *Preventing Physician Burnout* would be a mere shell of its current self without their nuanced and varied perspectives.

We extend our thanks and gratitude to our families. Paul would like to thank his wife, Bonnie, and children, Anna and Rosie. Diane would like to thank her husband, Sam, and children, Alexandra, Kira, and Niall. Without their support we might not have survived our bouts with burnout and regained the stamina and resilience required to advocate for change.

# DEDICATION

*We dedicate this book to the thousands of physicians affected by burnout, to our colleagues lost to suicide, and to their families. We also dedicate this book to the health care leaders who are trying to understand the causes of burnout and how best to create positive change in the health care workplace, and to patients, who deserve to be cared for by physicians at their best.*

# FOREWORD

B urnout is a hot topic in today's workplace, given its high costs for both employees and organizations. Within health care, these outcomes include such things as poor quality of patient care and more medical errors. When physicians and nurses are experiencing higher levels of burnout, their patients are less satisfied with the care they are receiving and are at a greater risk for patient mortality. Burnout is also linked to dysfunctional relationships with colleagues and with a stronger intention to leave the medical profession altogether. And like all experiences of stress, burnout can lead to poor physical health, family problems, greater substance abuse, and a higher risk of depression and suicidal ideation.

The urgency for addressing burnout arises not simply from the discomfort inherent in the experience but from all these other serious consequences in the workplace. It is not simply that "physicians are having a bad day" (and therefore it is their own personal problem). The research evidence indicates that burnout does not arise simply as a personal failing. Rather, burnout develops in response to problematic relationships between people and their workplaces and is therefore a social and organizational issue. When that workplace does not recognize the human side of work and there are major mismatches between the nature of the job and the nature of people, then there will be a greater risk of burnout.

What is exciting about this new book, *Preventing Physician Burnout*, is that Paul DeChant and Diane Shannon clearly recognize this job-person interface of burnout and have tackled it directly. Both of them each have the professional qualifications and the personal experience to understand the critical issues that burnout poses for the health care system. And DeChant and Shannon take the next important step of not only sharing their insights but actually proposing effective solutions, based on their work with Lean. This book has many valuable lessons to be learned and applied, by organizations that want to do something to reduce the risk of physician burnout. It provides the evidence for a better path in health care as well as the personal guidance for restoring passion and joy to the practice of medicine.

Christina Maslach, PhD
University of California, Berkeley

# INTRODUCTION

*I feel beaten down, exhausted, overwhelmed. I wake up in
the middle of the night, feeling the weight of this enormous
responsibility, because I know things fall through the
cracks. And there is so much administrative work—order
entry, billing entry. It just never ends. There is no quiet
minute to think about the patient. I think physicians are
at the breaking point. I'm looking for a way to leave.*
—PHYSICIAN IN HIS MID-40S

This book is an urgent call to action.

The crisis of physician burnout impacts virtually every health care organization in the country. Recent studies indicate that more than half of all physicians report at least one symptom of burnout—a figure has grown significantly in just the past few years. (Shanafelt 2015) The dedicated physicians in this country need solutions to fix the substantial problems in the current work environment.

Researchers have shown that professional burnout results from a mismatch between the worker and the workplace that harms the worker. (Maslach 2001) When more than half of physicians are burned out, the problem is not the worker—it's the work environment. External forces are increasingly changing the workplace in ways that create barriers and frustrations to providing patient care with the quality and empathy to which physicians aspire. The time has come for health care leaders to partner with physicians to manage the impact of those external forces and create a healthy work environment.

The experience of practicing medicine has become unsustainable. Physicians are cutting back on clinical practice, leaving practice entirely, or continuing to practice but in a disillusioned, disengaged state. The negative consequences of this epidemic for physicians, patients, health care organizations, clinical and non-clinical staff, and our communities are far reaching.

As a nation, we cannot fix our broken health care system without addressing burnout. Health care organizations cannot navigate the multitude of changes in our current delivery system without a cadre of fully engaged, energized physicians. The promise of technological innovations and the expansion of the health care workforce with nurse practitioners and physician assistants will fall far short of their potential to curb burnout without the leadership of engaged physicians.

Physician burnout and job dissatisfaction are among the most common topics in forums on physician-frequented websites, such as KevinMD, and are increasingly discussed in the lay press and peer-reviewed journals.

Despite this attention in the media, too many leaders of health care organizations remain unaware of the extent of the problem, its actual root causes, and its downstream negative effects on critical performance metrics of their organization.

An increasing number of leaders are addressing burnout by implementing physician wellness programs and offering burnout coaches. These are absolutely vital services that help many physicians cope who otherwise would be suffering.

Although this approach treats the symptoms of burnout, these programs do not change the underlying root cause of the problem: highly motivated and mission-driven professionals are working in toxic work environments in which they are unable to succeed.

The current situation is nobody's fault. The system has evolved over decades during which there have been numerous changes in reimbursement models and regulatory policies, substantial shifts in patient demographics, and advances in technology and treatment. All this change has occurred without intentional work to alter management approaches or workflow processes. What once worked fairly well is now failing miserably.

Although this situation is nobody's fault, it is every stakeholder's responsibility to do his or her part to fix the problem. Health care leaders and frontline physicians must work together to effect real change.

Too commonly, individual physicians are seen as the cause of the problem—they are "dinged" for being disengaged, uncooperative, and unaligned with important organizational goals. Looking only at these secondary symptoms of burnout, leaders (and physicians themselves) fail to see the true drivers of burnout today—the multiple barriers and frustrations clinicians face on a daily basis in their efforts to provide high-quality care and forge healing relationships with their patients.

Leaders must understand these drivers because leadership plays a critical role in fixing the root causes of burnout—and failure to do so exposes the organization to a multitude of downstream negative consequences. We will discuss the underlying drivers of physician burnout in more detail in Part 2.

In addition, although the prevalence and possible causes of physician burnout have been widely discussed in the media and in academic literature, proven strategies for *preventing* physician burnout are in short supply.

This is the reason we wrote *Preventing Physician Burnout*. We are passionate about preventing physician burnout, because it has touched us personally, and we have seen firsthand the harm it is causing our colleagues and our profession.

## WHO WE ARE

Paul is a family physician who moved into administration to help fix the toxic work environments he experienced in full-time practice. He believed that he could improve the leadership of health care organizations by focusing on the Lean principle of Respect for People. After 25 years as a practicing family physician and 30 years of progressive management experience, he is now an executive coach and consultant with Simpler Healthcare, an IBM Watson Health affiliate with a long history of supporting organizations through Lean transformations.

Diane is an internist who left practice after just three years because of burnout and dismay about her future career. She has been a freelance health care writer for 17 years, focusing on improvement strategies to address the issues that curtailed her clinical career.

Today, we feel more strongly than ever the urgency of the need to address physician burnout. While serving as CEO of a 300-physician medical group, Paul led the group through a Lean transformation. Struck by the degree of frustration, disengagement, and burnout he observed among the physicians, he chose to focus that transformation on the theme of "Returning Joy to Patient Care." Having experienced the power of that transformation to improve the lives of physicians, patients, support staff, and leaders, he is now focused on helping others develop a work environment in which physicians can achieve the vision they held when beginning medical school—one in which all physicians thrive, collaborate with patients, and partner with health care leaders in a supportive environment.

Diane first wrote publicly about her experience with burnout and leaving practice in an online post for WBUR, the Boston National Public Radio affiliate. She was shocked by the number of physicians who contacted her after reading the piece and by the poignancy of the stories of those she later interviewed. One physician wrote:

Hope you don't mind an e-mail from a stranger, but I recently read your article, and I wanted to send you a big thank-you. I went into medicine for the right reasons but find myself, after only six years, approaching burnout. Much of what you wrote are thoughts that I have had but felt like I would be a failure if I were to ever actually say them out loud. On a daily basis, I face all four of the factors associated with higher burnout. I feel frustrated by the lack of support from the administration. I'm very grateful to know that I'm not alone in these thoughts, and I really appreciate your words.

Another physician sent a similar comment:

I have recently come across your article about physician burnout when I Googled, "Why do physicians hate their job so much?"

And how you describe your anxiety, the inability to stop thinking about the patients, the need to micromanage and double-check everything, it rang so true to me that I was sure you were inside my thoughts. I'm a 47-year-old pediatric specialist, and I feel like I am too old and experienced to still be afraid of my job, but I am. The worst part is, I didn't feel like there's anyone else out there who's experiencing this until I read your article. This must be the dirty secret of medicine. It's good to hear I am not alone. Just wish I had a quick exit plan.

In talking with these physicians one on one, Diane heard both urgency and conflict in their voices—their strong desire to continue being caregivers and their simultaneous desperation to leave.

## OUR MISSION

Our mission is to correct physicians' and health care leaders' misperceptions about burnout and about how best to treat and prevent it. We also want to correct their misperceptions about Lean, because we firmly believe that Lean, when done right, can prevent physician burnout.

The voices of discouraged, disheartened, and despairing physicians have propelled both of us to think deeply about the problem and its prevention, to seek out the opinions of experts in relevant fields, and, finally, to put into words our thinking about the problem and a solution. The result of this quest is a deeply held belief that Lean, when done right, can prevent burnout by eliminating the daily barriers and frustrations in clinical practice.

However, our quest has also shown us the importance of a clear and common understanding of what Lean entails. Lean is often misconstrued as being simply a set of tools for increasing efficiency. This false belief is understandable, because Lean is far too often implemented as a set of efficiency tools and nothing more.

Herein lies the problem. When people see Lean solely as a tool kit, they fail to consider two of its essential components: a structured, ongoing management system and—especially important in preventing burnout—the underlying principle of respect for the workforce. We use the term *Lean Done Right* to describe a management approach that is based on respect for people and that empowers frontline doctors and nurses to call attention to and craft workable solutions to eliminate the problems that "poke you every day," as one physician we interviewed put it.

In this book we will show how Lean Done Right can eliminate these pokes.

*We limit our attention in Preventing Physician Burnout to burnout among physicians, because our personal experience and professional observations have been focused on burnout in doctors. We are acutely aware, however, that the problem affects many other health care professionals. We strongly support efforts to understand and address burnout within these other groups. We also believe that our recommended prevention strategies will help mitigate the factors that lead to burnout in all clinicians.*

*We also recognize that clinicians are not the only professionals in health care who are experiencing burnout. Leadership has become increasingly more difficult in the new health care arena, and the turnover rate for health care executives is at an all-time high.*

We firmly believe that Lean, with its emphasis on positive leadership and organizational culture, respect for the frontline clinician, and an effective ongoing management system, can prevent burnout and return joy to the practice of medicine.

## THE STRUCTURE OF THIS BOOK

This book is divided into three sections. Part 1 defines burnout in Chapter 1 and describes its downstream effects in Chapter 2. In Part 2 we provide an in-depth survey of the underlying drivers of physician burnout. We show that its root causes originate from three levels—the individual, the workplace, and the external environment; we describe these root causes in chapters 3 through 8.

You may find that Parts 1 and 2 have a somewhat academic tone, because we describe and refer to the research that exists on many of the topics covered in these sections. Part 3, which explains our approach for preventing physician burnout, is rather different. Little evidence exists regarding the effectiveness of interventions to address physician burnout. Given the dearth of published literature, we developed our proposed approach based on our experience and that of an array of experts from the fields of burnout, Lean, and health care delivery. We begin Chapter 9 by describing the existing approaches to addressing burnout that are aimed at the individual physician. In Chapter 10, we provide, through a collection of vignettes, examples of the good work that many leaders are doing in their organizations to address burnout. In Chapter 11, we explain Lean management, show how Lean Done Right differs from commonly held conceptions of Lean, and demonstrate how Lean Done Right can prevent physician burnout. In Chapter 12, we lay out clear action steps that executive leaders, boards of directors, and physicians can take to prevent burnout.

We believe that these strategies can do more than simply alleviate burnout—we believe they can fix much of what ails health care.

## REFERENCES

Maslach C, Schaufeli WB, Leiter MP. Job burnout. *Annu Rev Psychol.* 2001;52:397–422.

Shanafelt TD, Hasan O, Dyrbye LN, Sinsky C, Satele D, Sloan J, West CP. Changes in burnout and satisfaction with work-life balance in physicians and the general US working population between 2011 and 2014. *Mayo Clin Proc.* 2015;90(12):1600–1613.

# PART 1

## UNDERSTANDING PHYSICIAN BURNOUT

The media is filled with first-person stories, research reports, and editorials proclaiming that physician burnout has reached a crisis level. Every day, physicians post moving personal anecdotes, and experts post their theories about why physicians are retiring early, cutting back on clinical hours, or leaving clinical practice entirely. Many blame the advent of electronic health records.

At the same time, physicians are criticized for making "lifestyle" choices if they select a specialty or a particular practice setting because it offers a better work-life balance. Their negative feedback is sometimes described as whining. They are sometimes seen by the lay public as highly paid professionals who have no cause for complaint.

What is going on in the world of physicians today? Is the trend we're witnessing a true phenomenon or just a glut of fatigued physicians? Has the media overstated the prevalence of physician burnout, or is it as commonplace as the stories have led us to believe?

In Part 1, we will define and describe physician burnout, creating a foundation from which to understand the many drivers of the problem and the potential solutions. In Chapter 1, we provide a definition for *burnout* and describe its three primary symptoms. We also discuss the data on the prevalence of burnout among physicians. In Chapter 2, we cover the consequences and costs—financial and human—associated with physician burnout.

# CHAPTER 1

## WHAT IS BURNOUT?

*Statistics about burnout can be misleading. There's a lot that they don't show, because doctors don't like to admit to burnout, especially when they're going through it. They don't know who to trust. It's like asking a patient how much he or she drinks. They are going to minimize it.*
—MICHELLE MUDGE-RILEY, DO, MHA,
CAREER COACH FOR PHYSICIANS

*Initially I was oblivious to burnout. I thought it was just resistance to change, but over the last four to five years I have come to believe it is real and it is deep.*
—ROBERT WACHTER, MD, PROFESSOR AND CHAIR, DEPARTMENT OF MEDICINE, UNIVERSITY OF CALIFORNIA, SAN FRANCISCO, AND AUTHOR OF *THE DIGITAL DOCTOR: HOPE, HYPE, AND HARM AT THE DAWN OF MEDICINE'S COMPUTER AGE*

### WHAT BURNOUT FEELS LIKE

*Paul's Story*

I've spent my career trying to fix dysfunctional workflows in clinical settings. When I first started this work in the early 1980s, I was completely unfamiliar with Lean, but I knew there had to be a way to reduce the barriers and frustrations I experienced as I tried to take care of my patients.

Over the course of my career, I've experienced the classic symptoms of burnout—exhaustion, cynicism, and a sense of inefficacy.

During my 25 years of clinical practice as a family physician, I occasionally experienced burnout. At times in the middle of a busy day, when yet another patient was telling me about his or her seemingly unresolvable psychosocial problems while the waiting room piled up with more patients to see, I found myself fanaticizing about excusing myself from the room, getting in my car, and driving as far away as I could.

During my 30 years of progressive responsibility in management roles within health care organizations, which culminated in five years as CEO of a 300-physician medical group, I experienced burnout from the stress of needing to make and act on challenging leadership decisions. To cope, I found myself closing the door to my office over lunch so that no one else would bother me with yet another problem.

I learned to deal with the clinical burnout by working more closely in teams and collaborating with my partners and support staff. By helping each other, we managed to get through each day. But with the advent of the electronic health record (EHR), the work became much more intense, and it was harder to stave off burnout no matter how much our teams collaborated.

Leadership burnout was another story. As a change agent, I faced many significant challenges, including personal attacks from people I had regarded as peers aligned with me around a common purpose. It took a combination of my deep commitment to fixing health care, a willingness to step back and listen more carefully to people's concerns, and the support of good executive coaches and like-minded colleagues to get through the tough times. In retrospect, I know that I made plenty of mistakes along the way. And at least a couple of my moves—professional and geographical—were likely prompted by finding the situation I was in nearly intolerable.

Although there have been challenges along the way, the opportunity to positively impact the lives of my patients and of the physicians and support staff in the organizations I led made the journey worthwhile.

### Diane's Story
As a medical student and a resident in internal medicine, I loved patient contact and received stellar evaluations. I had no trouble with certifying

exams or my board exams in internal medicine, but I found the clinical environment jarring, harsh, and unsupportive. As a resident I often felt a sense of impending doom. I had the sense that the larger system in which I was working had major flaws and was not set up to catch mistakes before they harmed a patient. I felt I needed to be superhuman and always vigilant. I had trouble leaving work at work.

When I was a resident, I felt utter fatigue from the long hours, the sleep deprivation, and the effort of trying to make complex decisions when I was physically and mentally depleted. A five-year relationship ended, because I had nothing left to give. I often forgot ZIP codes and phone numbers I had known my whole life. Somehow, though, I managed to remember specific details about my patients, such as their serum potassium level and the status of their CT scan. Although I consider myself a compassionate person, during residency I found myself joining in with my colleagues in joking about our more difficult patients. I remember the dark humor that swirled around the halls during the bleak nights of training. Joking about our circumstances helped us avoid feeling completely overwhelmed by what we were doing and experiencing.

Despite overwhelming positive feedback from my mentors during residency, I often doubted my abilities and my judgment. I worried a lot about making mistakes, especially in an environment that demanded perfection yet seemed so broken. I hid my growing distress. I didn't feel that help was an option. I felt I needed to cope on my own.

After residency, I worked in several ambulatory settings, trying to find a practice in which I could thrive. I never did. I was discouraged when I looked ahead at my potential career and the life I thought I would have. I began to consider leaving, but I felt trapped, stressed, and confused. Who would I be if I weren't a physician? It was a really dark time. I knew I would miss patient contact if I left. I felt grief at the loss of a dream, grief for the loss of a profession I had hoped to have. But eventually I ran out of energy. I was worn down from pushing myself so hard, and I was losing touch with the reason I had entered the profession. Eventually I realized that I just couldn't do it anymore.

I was fortunate to be able to land on my feet. I transitioned to a non-clinical position and eventually launched a career as a freelance health care writer. Although my experience with burnout is now almost two decades in the past, the difficult memories, painful thoughts, and many losses remain. I've moved beyond burnout to craft a new life, but I haven't left it entirely behind.

## THE SYMPTOMS OF BURNOUT

Burnout consists of three symptoms: emotional exhaustion, depersonalization, and inefficacy. (Maslach 2001; Maslach 2008) *Emotional exhaustion* is the feeling of being overextended and depleted of one's emotional and physical resources. Recently, some researchers have begun favoring the term *exhaustion* alone to identify the cognitive and physical aspects of burnout.

Researchers have described the symptom as follows: (Maslach 2001)

> Exhaustion is not something that is simply experienced— rather, it prompts actions to distance oneself emotionally and cognitively from one's work, presumably as a way to cope with the work overload. Within the human services, the emotional demands of the work can exhaust a service provider's capacity to be involved with, and responsive to, the needs of service recipients. Depersonalization is an attempt to put distance between oneself and service recipients by actively ignoring the qualities that make them unique and engaging people.

The second symptom, *depersonalization*, or cynicism, is a negative, excessively detached, or callous response to one's job; among physicians, this symptom may present as distancing from patients. This symptom is a natural response to exhaustion. It is a coping mechanism for dealing with the sometimes overwhelming emotional stress inherent in service occupations. According to researchers, detachment is a way for the worker to protect him- or herself from intense emotional distress that might interfere with work effectiveness. By controlling the degree of compassion he or she feels for the person served and obtaining some emotional distance, the caregiver achieves a state of "detached concern." (Maslach 2001)

When physicians develop depersonalization, they may relate to patients in a dehumanized, callous way. Samuel Shem's fictionalized account of internship, *House of God*, illustrates well this detachment and cynicism. Clearly, depersonalization and callousness are antithetical to providing compassionate care, yet they are a predictable response to chronic emotional exhaustion.

The third symptom of burnout, *inefficacy*, manifests as a sense of reduced personal accomplishment and achievement at work, low productivity at one's job, and feelings of incompetence. Exhaustion and depersonalization can lead to inefficacy, as the first two symptoms interfere with a worker's effectiveness at his or her job. As researchers describe it, the sense of lower accomplishment is directly related to the other symptoms of burnout: "A work situation with chronic, overwhelming demands that contribute to exhaustion or cynicism is likely to erode one's sense of effectiveness." (Maslach 2001) Individuals who are drawn to a helping profession will not feel a great sense of accomplishment, or find joy and meaning in work if they feel emotionally depleted and indifferent to the people they are working to help.

Just as burnout has a specific definition, it also has a specific and validated tool for its measurement. Developed by Christina Maslach, PhD, professor emerita in the Department of Psychology at the University of California, Berkeley, in the 1970s, the Maslach Burnout Inventory (MBI) is widely used today to measure burnout among physicians. (Maslach 1981; Schaufeli 1996) However, as we learned in an interview with Dr. Maslach, the MBI was developed for research rather than for clinical use, and the tool does not assess or identify underlying causes of burnout (see the box titled "Measuring Burnout: Research versus Diagnosis").

---

## MEASURING BURNOUT: RESEARCH VERSUS DIAGNOSIS
**By Christina Maslach, PhD**

The MBI was developed as a research instrument—a tool for assessing the burnout experience and exploring its relationship to other factors (such as potential causes, outcomes, or correlates of burnout). Burnout is assessed on a continuum, ranging from low to high, on three different dimensions: emotional exhaustion, depersonalization, and reduced personal accomplishment. For example, it can be used to assess the patterns of burnout within groups of physicians. But the MBI must be used with other research tools in order to answer questions about why burnout occurs, how it develops or changes over time, and what interventions are effective in reducing its risk or preventing it.

However, the research perspective of a continuum is fundamentally different from that of a practitioner who views burnout as a discrete state—either someone is burned out or the person is not. The perspective that burnout is a dichotomy makes it more like a medical disease, rather than a continuum of experience. And it has led people to want a measure that will provide a dichotomous "diagnosis" of burnout.

The challenge has been to identify how to translate the continuous scores of a research measure into a dichotomous burnout classification. As an analogy, what is the temperature on a continuous thermometer scale that signals the presence or absence of fever? For burnout, what is the pattern of MBI scores that predict certain diagnostic criteria (such as impaired work performance, or absenteeism, or poor health)? Unfortunately, such diagnostic criteria have not been well specified, so the necessary clinical research has not been done. However, researchers in the Netherlands have used work-related neurasthenia as the equivalent of clinical burnout and have established that high scores on two of the burnout dimensions (exhaustion plus one other) are correlated with high scores on neurasthenia.

Another approach has been to use arbitrary, statistical "cutoff" scores to identify people who are "high" on burnout. For example, the MBI Manual reports the distribution of scores for its normative samples, by dividing them into thirds of "low," "average," and "high." Although useful for assessing the overall pattern of a group, such arbitrary "cutoff" scores do not have any diagnostic validity. In other words, the upper third of a large population is not a definition of people experiencing a severe case of burnout. A different approach has been to simplify the MBI assessment by using only the exhaustion dimension or by reducing the number of questions to only a few. However, this simplification runs the risk of converting the phenomenon of burnout into exhaustion alone and ignoring the relevance of depersonalization and professional inefficacy.

———

## THE OPPOSITE OF BURNOUT

In recent years, in part due to the greater recognition of burnout among physicians, a great deal of attention has been focused on restoring joy to practice. Since the first descriptions of burnout, research on the subject has focused on the negative and on ways to restore an individual to a neutral position (that is, not experiencing burnout). What about the positive, though? Studies of effective organizations have demonstrated the value of cultivating behaviors that are distinctly positive (referred to in psychology research as the positive deviance) rather than simply the absence of the negative. (Cameron 2003)

Dr. Maslach and colleagues have conducted preliminary studies regarding the positive—polar opposite of burnout. (Maslach 2011) They refer to this state as "work engagement." Its three dimensions correspond with the three symptoms of burnout (see figure 1).

We believe that the three "symptoms" of work engagement reflect a state that is necessary for physician job satisfaction, joy in practice, and engagement with their organization.

## RECOGNIZING BURNOUT IN YOUR ORGANIZATION

Leaders may overlook symptoms of burnout among the physicians in their organization for a number of reasons. After all, physicians tend to mask their distress (more on this in Chapter 4) and are unlikely to approach leaders or the board to request help for the problem. The last

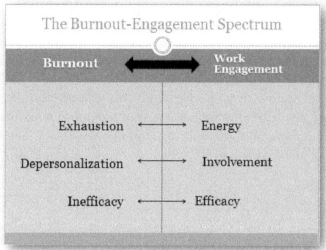

**Figure 1: The Burnout-Engagement Spectrum**
*Source*: Maslach 2011.

thing physicians are likely to do is openly display what they perceive to be a weakness or liability, especially to organizational leaders.

However, leaders who are not aware of physician burnout in their organization may recognize these secondary signs of the problem:

- High staff and physician turnover
- Vacant positions and difficulty recruiting physicians
- Disruptive physician behavior and angry complaints about consultants and nursing staff (and vice versa)
- Lack of physician engagement in strategic projects or improvement work
- Flat refusal to see additional patients
- Lack of attendance at medical staff meetings (in the past 300 physicians showed up; now meetings hover at about 50 participants)
- Angry complaints about electronic health records, quality metrics, the challenges of implementing best practices, open-access scheduling, and yet another improvement initiative
- Bitter protests that low patient satisfaction scores are beyond their control
- Demands from frustrated physicians for compensation for everything they do

When frustrated physicians complain about a new improvement initiative or technology upgrade, when they balk at a new policy or resist the attempts of administration to engage them as champions, and when they react with negativity to any and all feedback about their performance, leaders may be tempted to label their difficult behavior as "whining."

Burnout is not whining. Although it may present as difficult, disruptive, or undermining behavior, burnout is not simply the dissatisfaction of highly paid professionals bitterly resisting change. Burnout is a predictable response to chronic stress that has negative psychological, physical, and cognitive effects. These negative effects take a toll on physicians, on their patients, and on the metrics most important to organizational leaders, including quality, safety, productivity, patient satisfaction, and cost.

## THE PREVALENCE OF PHYSICIAN BURNOUT

It seems as though talk about the "epidemic" of physician burnout is everywhere—from influential health care groups, such as the American Medical Association, the American College of Physicians, and the Institute for Healthcare Improvement, to the lay press, including *The Huffington Post*, *The Atlantic*, and *The New Yorker*. The media is rife with stories about the widespread prevalence of burnout among doctors, but just how pervasive is the problem? It is, in fact, both widespread and increasing.

A 2014 survey by Tait Shanafelt, MD, and his colleagues at the Mayo Clinic found that more than half of almost 7,000 physicians surveyed reported one or more symptoms of burnout. (Shanafelt 2015) The average across all specialties was 54 percent, up from 45 percent in 2011, representing an almost 10 percent increase in just three years. (Shanafelt 2015) In addition, reported satisfaction with work-life balance had declined significantly for physicians over the same three-year time period, from 48 percent in 2011 to 41 percent in 2014. Burnout was present in all 24 specialties studied and had increased by 10 percent or more over three years in 9 of those specialties.

Notably, burnout and work-life balance in the comparison group, that is, individuals with professional careers, remained unchanged (and was substantially better than for physicians). In fact, the risk of burnout for physicians is twice as great as the risk among the general population. (Shanafelt 2015)

Previous studies substantiate these numbers. A 2008 study of almost 8,000 US surgeons found a burnout rate of 40 percent. (Shanafelt 2009) In a 2009 study of more than 2,600 medical students, 53 percent reported symptoms of burnout. (Dyrbye 2010) The 2016 annual Medscape survey, which included responses from almost 16,000 physicians, found an average burnout rate ranging from 40 to 55 percent, depending on the specialty. (Medscape 2016) Rates were higher than in 2015 for every one of the 25 specialties polled. On the flip side, when asked in the most recent Medscape poll whether they were happy at work, the proportion of physicians reporting that they were very or extremely happy ranged from just 24 percent for internists to 39 percent for dermatologists. (Medscape 2016)

In a 2015 online survey conducted by the executive search firm Cejka Search, 88 percent of the approximately 2,000 physicians that responded reported, on a 10-point Likert scale, being moderately to severely stressed or burned out on an average day, and 46 percent reported severe stress or burnout. (VITAL WorkLife and Cejka Search 2016) (Note that, unlike the other studies mentioned, this survey did not use the MBI to assess burnout.)

In addition, markers of career satisfaction indicate that most physicians are not happy with their work life these days. A 2012 online survey of more than 7,000 physicians found that just 1 in 10 would recommend the profession as a career. (Doctors Company 2012) Another study from the same year found that more than half of the surveyed primary care physicians aged 50 or older planned to leave practice within five years. (Gray 2012) Even more alarming, 30 percent of the primary care physicians age 35 to 39 also indicated that they planned to leave clinical practice within five years.

The Mayo Clinic study also found a reduction in satisfaction with work-life balance among physicians between the 2011 and 2014 studies (from 48.5% to 40.9%, P< 0.001). The authors noted that "substantial erosion in satisfaction with work-life balance has…been observed among US physicians over the past 3 years, despite no increase in the median number of hours worked per week." (Shanafelt 2015)

Burnout prevalence varies to some degree based on physician characteristics, such as specialty, years in practice, age, and gender. According to the Mayo Clinic study, in 2014 the 10 specialties with the highest rates of reported burnout were: (Shanafelt 2015)

- Emergency medicine
- Urology
- Physical medicine and rehabilitation
- Family medicine
- Radiology
- Orthopedic surgery
- Dermatology
- General surgery subspecialties
- Pathology
- General pediatrics

The Medscape survey, based on 2015 data, found that the following specialties had the highest rates of burnout: (Medscape 2016)

- Emergency medicine (55%)
- Critical care medicine (55%)
- Urology (55%)
- Family medicine (54%)
- Internal medicine (54%)
- Pediatrics (53%)
- Surgery (52%)
- Obstetrics-Gynecology (51%)
- Neurology (51%)
- Radiology (50%)

The number of years in practice also appears to affect the risk of burnout, with young physicians (less than 35 years of age) at greatest risk for burnout and for dissatisfaction with work-life balance. (Shanafelt 2015) (These data corroborate Diane's experience: the majority of physicians who contact her to ask advice or share their stories of burnout are in training or within the first five years of practice. Of course, that may reflect a selection bias related to those physicians who have the time and inclination to ask for help in this way.)

Many studies have documented an increased prevalence of reported burnout among female physicians. For example, a 2016 study of primary care physicians found a higher rate of burnout among female doctors (36% vs. 19%). (Rabatin 2016) In the most recent Medscape survey, 55 percent of female physicians reported being burned out, compared with 46 percent of their male counterparts. (Medscape 2016) The Mayo Clinic data demonstrated a statistically significant increased risk of burnout among female physicians compared with their male colleagues. (Shanafelt 2015)

Experts have offered a number of hypotheses about the reasons for this disparity, including greater family responsibilities for women (Moukas 2003), and the tendency for patients to expect more in-depth conversations with female physicians, which adds to the time pressure they experience (personal communication, Mark Linzer, MD, June 27, 2016). Alternately, as Mudge-Riley pointed out when we interviewed her, male physicians might be less likely to report burnout symptoms or may report different symptoms. Her practice includes an equal number of male and female clients.

Despite these variations among certain groups, burnout cuts across every demographic and exists in every subpopulation of physicians. Indeed, burnout is more prevalent in physicians than in the general US working population, even after adjusting for age, sex, relationship status, and hours worked per week. (Shanafelt 2015)

No physician, it seems, is immune to burnout—not even those who attain highly respected leadership positions in prestigious health care organizations. Gene Lindsey, MD, former president and CEO of Atrius Health, a large health system in Boston, described his personal experience with burnout in an interview: "I felt uncertain inside, insecure about my abilities. My patients had become a hassle that prevented me from leaving. I felt like a deficient human being. I felt depressed. At one point I was almost suicidal. Fortunately, in an attempt to rescue myself, I sought counseling."

♫♫♫

Why is the scope of physician burnout so important? Because, as we describe in Chapter 2, the associated costs and consequences of burnout among doctors—to individuals and to health care organizations—are substantial.

## REFERENCES

Cameron KS, Dutton JE, Quinn RE. *Positive Organizational Scholarship.* San Francisco: Berrett-Koehler. 2003.

The Doctors Company Market Research. The future of health care: a national survey of physicians. 2012. Available at: http://www.thedoctors.com/TDC/Pressroom/CON_ID_004672?refId=FUTURE. Accessed February 2, 2016.

Dyrbye LN, Massie FS, Jr, Eacker A, Harper W, Power D, Durning SJ. Relationship between burnout and professional conduct and attitudes among US medical students. *JAMA.* 2010;(304):1173–1180.

Gray BH, Stockley K, Zuckerman S. American primary care physicians' decisions to leave their practice: evidence from the 2009 commonwealth fund survey of primary care doctors. *J Prim Care Community Health.* 2012;3(3):187–194.

Leiter MP, Maslach C. A mediation model of job burnout. In: Antoniou, A-S B, Cooper CL, eds. *Research Companion to Organizational Health Psychology.* Northampton, MA: Edward Elgar Publishing Inc. 2005.

Maslach C. Commentary: engagement research: some thoughts from a burnout perspective. *Eur J Work Organ Psy.* 2011;20(1):47–52.

Maslach C, Goldberg C. Prevention of burnout: new perspectives. *Appl Prevent Psychol.* 1998;7:63–74.

Maslach C, Jackson SE. The measurement of experienced burnout. *J Occ Behav.* 1996;2:99–113.

Maslach C, Leiter MP. Early predictors of job burnout and engagement. *J Appl Psychol.* 2008;93(3):498–512.

Maslach C, Schaufeli WB, Leiter MP. Job burnout. *Annu Rev Psychol.* 2001;52:397–422.

Medscape. Medscape lifestyle report 2016: bias and burnout. Available at: http://www.medscape.com/features/slideshow/lifestyle/2016/public/overview. Accessed February 4, 2016.

Moukas E, Davidson A, Kaufmann V. OMA Physician Health Program explores help-seeking behaviours of women physicians. *Ont Med Rev.* 2003;70:41–43.

Rabatin J, Williams E, Baier Manwell L, Schwartz MD, Brown RL, Linzer M. Predictors and outcomes of burnout in primary care physicians. *J Prim Care Community Health.* 2016;7(1):41–43.

Schaufeli WB, Leiter MP, Maslach C, Jackson SE. The Maslach Burnout Inventory—general survey. In: Maslach C, Jackson SE, Leiter MP, eds. *MBI Manual.* 3rd ed. Palo Alto, CA: Consulting Psychologists Press. 1996.

Shanafelt TD, Balch CM, Bechamps GJ, et al. Burnout and career satisfaction among American surgeons. *Ann Surg.* 2009;250(3):463–471.

Shanafelt TD, Boone S, Tan L, et al. Burnout and satisfaction with work-life balance among US physicians relative to the general US population. *Arch Intern Med.* 2012;172:1377–1385.

Shanafelt TD, Hasan O, Dyrbye LN, et al. Changes in burnout and satisfaction with work-life balance in physicians and the general US working population between 2011 and 2014. *Mayo Clin Proc.* 2015;90(12):1600–1613.

VITAL WorkLife and Cejka Search. 2015 Physician Stress and Burnout Survey. 2016. Available at: http://info.vitalworklife.com/stress. Accessed April 21, 2016.

West CP, Shanafelt TD, Kolars JC. Quality of life, burnout, educational debt, and medical knowledge among internal medicine residents. *JAMA.* 2011;306(9):952–960.

# CHAPTER 2

## CONSEQUENCES OF PHYSICIAN BURNOUT

*Some physicians leave. They amputate themselves from the situation, cutting their losses. By removing the gangrenous foot, the rest of the body is spared. However, there is a net overall effect: loss to themselves, to their current patients, to any future patients, and to the possible contribution of a career well lived for all of humanity.*
—ERRIN WEISMAN, DO[1]

*As joy in the work force erodes, quality goes down.*
—DONALD BERWICK, MD, MPP, PRESIDENT EMERITUS AND SENIOR FELLOW, INSTITUTE FOR HEALTHCARE IMPROVEMENT[2]

- Are your physicians slow to engage in performance improvement initiatives?
- Does your organization struggle to fill open clinical positions?
- Is disruptive physician behavior a continuing problem?
- Does your hospital or practice suffer from high staff turnover?

---

1 Weisman E. This doctor quit medicine. It saved her life. [Internet]. Available at: http://www.kevinmd.com/blog/2016/03/doctor-quit-medicine-saved-life.html. Accessed July 8, 2016.
2 Institute for Healthcare Improvement. How does joy in work advance quality and safety? Available at: https://www.youtube.com/watch?v=3JTdHStR6KI. Accessed April 29, 2016.

- Have an increasing number of physicians in your organization quit, retired early, or reduced their clinical hours?
- Has a physician from your organization died by suicide in the recent past?

If you answered affirmatively to one or more of these questions, more likely than not your organization is experiencing the consequences of physician burnout. Burnout takes a toll on the affected physician and has a ripple effect on everyone in the health care system: other physicians, clinical and non-clinical staff, patients and their families, provider organizations and their leaders, health care payers, and employers.

Physician burnout can mask as disruptive behavior. Disruptive behavior often results when physicians react to perceived unfairness, frustrations in the work environment, or situations that jeopardize the quality of care they provide. Whatever the trigger, disruptive behavior is never justified. It puts patients, co-workers, and provider organizations at risk—and it deflects attention from the underlying problems that need to be addressed. Disruptive behavior also creates additional stress for the medical staff leaders, increasing their risk of burnout.

In an interview, Theresa Brown, RN, a hospice nurse, frequent contributor to the *New York Times*, and author of *The Shift: One Nurse, Twelve Hours, Four Patients' Lives*, described the effects of physician burnout on other clinicians: "Physicians are at the top of the food chain on patient care units. They have power and authority, so if they are burned out and display difficult behavior, if they are aggressive or don't answer pages, it has a trickle-down effect. The nurse gets frustrated and takes it out on the nurse's aide or the transport tech. If, instead, the physician is present, engaged, and glad to be at work, that has a positive trickle-down effect."

Brown also noted the effects of physician burnout on professionalism. She believes that physicians who are sarcastic, negative, or cavalier in their attitude or actions model that behavior for nurses and other clinicians rather than model the embrace of professionalism and the display of appropriate behavior, even when dealing with difficult patients. Brown pointed to the hidden costs of working with someone who is burned out, saying, "Health care is such a complex system that we need the wheels to turn smoothly. If you're working with someone who doesn't care or can't care because of depression or whatever they're dealing with, it makes everything harder."

Although many of the consequences of physician burnout are interwoven, for ease of discussion we will describe the effects on four groups: affected physicians, patients, health care organizations, and the larger health care system. Our choice of order is intentional, because burnout directly inhibits a physician's ability to provide high-quality, safe, compassionate care, which adversely affects his or her patients. These effects on patient care adversely impact the performance of health care organizations, which ultimately affects the cost, quality, safety, and availability of health care services at the societal level.

## THE EFFECTS OF BURNOUT ON AFFECTED PHYSICIANS

Burnout exacts a substantial personal toll on affected physicians. They experience disillusionment, stress, and confusion as they struggle to continue caring for others while being depleted themselves. The effects of burnout also spill out into the physician's family relationships and personal life. According to Wayne Sotile, PhD, author of *The Resilient Physician: Effective Emotional Management for Doctors and Their Medical Organizations* and founder of the Center for Physician Resilience, a wellness center for individual physicians and their families, the negative effects of burnout on the physician's personal life result in a downward spiral, and the physician eventually experiences stress and negativity both at work and at home.

As a result of burnout, many physicians cut back on clinical practice or leave practice entirely. Dissatisfied physicians are two times more likely to cut back on or leave practice within two years than are their more satisfied colleagues. (Landon 2003) Burned-out physicians are more likely than their colleagues to report an intention to leave their current position within the next 36 months, to decrease work hours, or to leave patient care entirely. (Shanafelt 2009 archives; Rabatin 2016)

For Diane and for the physicians with burnout we interviewed, the decision to leave practice was extremely difficult and not taken lightly. As a hospitalist told us, "People who get all the way through medical training are not quitters, so leaving was an additional struggle. But at some point, I just thought, 'Get me out of here.'" Most eventually made peace with the decision, but they had a keen awareness of the personal losses associated with leaving their chosen profession.

Physician distress can have dire consequences if untreated. A study of surgeons found that those who were burned out or depressed were significantly more likely to suffer from alcohol abuse or dependence. (Oreskovich 2012) Physicians die by suicide at a rate much higher than the general population. In a study of more than 4,000 medical students, burnout was an independent predictor of suicidal ideation over the subsequent year. (Dyrbye 2008) Of the students who met the criteria for burnout, about 27 percent had recovered when assessed one year later. Recovery was associated with substantially less suicide ideation. A meta-analysis documented that female physicians have a suicide rate that is 130 percent higher than that of women in the general population. (Schernhammer 2004) The rate for male physicians is about 40 percent higher than for men in the general population. In fact, the death rate of physicians is lower than that of the general population for every major cause of death, including coronary artery disease, stroke, cancer, and respiratory disease, with the exception of suicide, for which it is substantially higher. (Torre 2005)

Pamela Wible, MD, founder of the Ideal Medical Care Movement and the 2015 American Medical Student Association Woman Leader in Medicine, became the leading voice for addressing the impact of physician suicide after realizing the impact in her own small community: "I was sitting at the memorial service for the third physician that we had lost to suicide [in 18 months] in my small town. I was sitting behind his five children and his wife. I started counting on my fingers the numbers of suspicious deaths and suicides among doctors that I knew about. In a very short period of time, I had used all 10 fingers. I was overwhelmed with the thought." She is concerned that the term *burnout* can be used as a label that shames and blames physicians, rather than as one that points to the root causes of burnout, which are the ways our training programs and workplace environments place physicians and trainees at risk.

Several possible explanations exist for physicians' heightened risk for suicide, including access to lethal means (that is, medications), the hesitancy of physicians to admit to symptoms that might affect their ability to practice or register as "weakness," and the tendency of physicians to diagnose and treat themselves. Starla Fitch, MD, is an oculoplastic surgeon who experienced and recovered from burnout. She continues to practice and is now a coach for physicians with burnout. According to Fitch, needing help still carries a stigma in medicine. "We don't want to say we don't know anything, let alone admit when we're in trouble."

Physicians' self-identity is often closely tied to their professional image, increasing their vulnerability to stress from problems at work. (Innelli 2014) Physician suicide victims are more likely than non-physician victims to have had a recent job problem. (Gold 2012)

Physician suicide victims also have a greater likelihood of mental illness, but a lower likelihood of antidepressant treatment than other suicide victims. (Gold 2012) At the same, physicians who die by their own hand are much more likely than other suicide victims to have drug levels of other psychoactive medications, including benzodiazepines, barbiturates, and antipsychotics. (Gold 2012)

Burnout also increases the risk of early death by traffic accidents. A 2012 study of residents found that burnout, depression, and fatigue were each significantly associated with the risk of a motor vehicle incident in the subsequent three months. (West 2012)

## THE EFFECTS OF BURNOUT ON PATIENT CARE

Patient outcomes are affected by many factors, only some of which are influenced by physicians. For this reason, it can be difficult to show a direct relationship between physician burnout and specific, objective patient outcomes. However, the collection of available evidence makes a compelling case for the adverse effects of burnout on patient care.

When we consider the three symptoms of burnout, it is logical that physician burnout would have direct consequences for patient care. A physician who is emotionally exhausted may be less likely to go the extra mile to have a difficult yet important conversation with a patient's family or to be exacting with recommended care practices. A physician experiencing depersonalization is unlikely to be as compassionate and empathetic as he or she might be otherwise. A physician who is struggling with inefficacy and doubting his or her performance or the meaning of the work may be unable to fully engage in change initiatives that would ultimately improve patient care. Presenteeism—being at work but not able to function fully because of illness or other medical conditions—is recognized as a major cause of lost productivity. (Hemp 2004) Physicians with burnout who continue to work epitomize the problem of presenteeism, because they are unable to perform at full capacity.

Recent research has identified a serious sequela of burnout that could directly affect patient care. Research psychologists have demonstrated that burnout is associated with a significant reduction in cognitive functioning and with changes in the brain that are visible with functional MRI. (Golkar 2016) In other studies, researchers have found that greater cognitive load due to stress has effects on brain functioning similar to those of alcohol, sleep deprivation, or a 13-point drop in IQ points. (Mani 2013) Having to consider all of the opportunity costs of each decision (as physicians under intense time and productivity pressure must do) increases cognitive load and thus may impact a physician's decision-making abilities.

As Dan Ariely, PhD, and William L. Lanier, MD, pointed out in a recent editorial in *Mayo Clinic Proceedings*, "Given [the] effects of cognitive scarcity, the negative implications of having to continually manage time as well as all the other difficult decisions that physicians faced should make physicians highly susceptible to cognitive exhaustion and, ultimately, poor quality decisions." (Ariely 2015) According to Maslach, data such as these show that burnout can have serious effects on a physician's health and cognitive functioning. This means that those organizational leaders who have deemed burnout a nuisance problem need to reconsider. As she told us, "Some leaders say, 'I am running a business here. So if people are having a bad day, and call that burnout, then that's their problem, not mine.'"

## Patient safety
Burnout has definitive effects on safety practices. In a study from the Mayo Clinic, about 9 percent of surgeons reported a major medical error within the prior three months, and surgeons who reported an error were

significantly more likely to have symptoms of burnout. (Shanafelt 2010) In addition, burnout and depression remained independent predictors of reporting a recent major medical error even after researchers controlled for other personal and professional factors. In fact, for each one-point increase on the depersonalization dimension of the Maslach Burnout Inventory, the likelihood of reporting an error increased by 11 percent.

Studies of trainees showed similar results. A 2008 study found an increased risk of medication errors among residents who were depressed or burned out. (Fahrenkopf 2008) A 2009 study demonstrated that residents who reported burnout symptoms were more likely to subsequently make self-reported medical errors; conversely, residents who made self-reported medical errors were more likely to screen positive for burnout in follow-up testing. (West 2006)

## Quality of care

In addition to its adverse effects on patient safety, burnout has demonstrable negative consequences on care quality. Jean E. Wallace, PhD, and her colleagues described the effects of burnout on quality in an article entitled "Physician Wellness: A Missing Quality Indicator," which was published in the The Lancet. "When physicians are unwell, the performance of health-care systems can be sub-optimum. Physician wellness might not only benefit the individual physician; it could also be vital to the delivery of high-quality health care." (Wallace 2009)

Burnout is indeed associated with reduced standards of care. A 2010 study showed that burnout among medical students was associated with self-reported unprofessional conduct and less altruistic professional values. (Dyrbye 2010)

In a 2002 study, residents with high scores for burnout were more likely to report suboptimal care practices, such as errors that were not due to inexperience or lack of knowledge. (Shanafelt 2002) A later study of primary care physicians found similar results. Researchers found that burnout was associated with a higher rate of self-reported likelihood of error and suboptimal patient care. (Linzer 2009) The study did not find an effect on standard quality and safety measures, however. Mark Linzer,

MD, director of the Division of General Internal Medicine at Hennepin County Medical Center and one of the study investigators, believes this reflects a buffer effect: "Physicians in stressful work environments work very hard to protect their patients from adverse effects that would be reflected in lower quality measures. They may preserve the outcome metrics, but at a high personal price."

Physicians are often aware of the negative effect on care practices, which may reflect the inefficacy component of burnout. In a 1997 study, one-third of physicians reported reduced standards of care, which they most commonly related to fatigue and work pressure. (Firth-Cozens 1997) A more recent study documented that physicians with burnout are more likely to consider themselves less capable of providing quality care. (Williams 2007) Similarly, among family physicians career dissatisfaction is associated with self-reported decreased ability to provide quality care. (Devoe 2002)

## Patient experience

Paul Grundy, MD, MPH, serves dual roles: global director of health care transformation for IBM and founding president of the Patient-Centered Primary Care Collaborative. He has written, "What patients want is that deep relationship with a healer. This is the foundation upon which we need to build health care." (Grundy 2016)

Consider a time when you or a family member needed medical care. How important was the tenor of your interactions with your care provider? How important was his or her ability to offer compassion, be empathetic, treat you with respect, and communicate clearly with you? Recalling this experience, you can appreciate the importance of a positive patient experience. Physician burnout adversely affects the physician-patient relationship and the experience of care. At an instinctual level, this makes sense. Physicians with emotional exhaustion or depersonalization are unlikely to be able to be fully present for others who are suffering. Because of the key role that frontline clinicians play in the care experience, personal interactions with physicians profoundly affect patients. A negative interaction makes a lasting impression.

Research on patient and physician satisfaction supports this assertion. Patient satisfaction with care closely correlates with physician career satisfaction within a given geographic region. (DeVoe 2007) A survey of more than 2,000 patients found that those whose physicians were very or extremely satisfied with their work reported greater overall satisfaction with their health care. (Haas 2000)

In addition to these demonstrated effects of physician burnout on the patient experience of care, patients also suffer when career dissatisfaction or burnout results in physicians leaving or cutting back on practice. Care continuity and ongoing therapeutic relationships suffer with increased physician turnover.

Meg Gaines, JD, LLM, distinguished clinical professor at the University of Wisconsin, is director of the Center for Patient Partnerships, which she co-founded in 2000 to provide advocacy for patients, motivated by her personal experience as a cancer patient. In an interview, Gaines articulated her view of the connection between care provider satisfaction and the patient experience.

> As a patient and patient advocate, I have absolutely no doubt that my care provider's health, well-being, and joy in work are inextricably linked to my health, well-being, and joy in life. A clinician who is unwell or unhappy will not be able to provide me with high-quality health care on a sustained basis. And he or she won't be able to help me make decisions that are consistent with my values, because doing so requires high-level emotional skills, like providing the right information, helping me clarify my values, and matching the available choices with my preference and my definition of quality of life. Skills like these take a lot of effort, which a dissatisfied, burned-out clinician is unlikely to summon consistently.

Burnout hinders a physician's ability to effectively use the skills that Gaines describes so eloquently and that are absolutely integral to an optimal patient experience. In contrast, physician engagement, which is unlikely to be present in burned-out physicians, correlates with a positive patient experience.

Brown also sees a direct connection between caregiver well-being and the patient experience: "In health care we set the bar low in terms of caregivers and how human we allow them to be—and it's a totally human job. We're trying to help sad, sick people get better. We're not making TV sets. We must honor our own humanity if we are to take care of that aspect of our patients."

Physician engagement has been shown to strongly correlate with patient engagement. Analysts for Press Ganey have found that health care organizations with higher scores on employee and physician engagement receive higher scores on patient experience surveys. (Press Ganey 2013) The difference is impressive: organizations that scored in the top decile in physician engagement had patient experience scores that were about 50 percent higher than those of the hospitals in the lowest decile for physician engagement.

## THE EFFECTS OF BURNOUT ON HEALTH CARE ORGANIZATIONS

Given the demonstrated effects of physician burnout on patient safety, care quality, and patient experience, an obvious conclusion is that the performance of health care organizations is at risk if their physicians are suffering from burnout. In addition to a dampening effect on the organization's quality and safety metrics, burnout is likely to affect its culture, finances, and overall performance and organizational resilience.

### Culture

Physician burnout and dissatisfaction have been shown to have adverse effects on the morale and organizational culture of health care organizations. (Misra-Hebert 2004) Physicians experiencing emotional exhaustion are unlikely to be able to deal as easily with communication issues involving colleagues or nursing staff. Relationships with colleagues, nursing staff, administrators, and other clinical and non-clinical staff are likely to suffer. Whether it is burnout per se or the stressors causing burnout that adversely affect organizational culture, the result is a work environment unconducive to the collaborative, team-based care needed to succeed under value-based payment models. Burnout, especially the symptom of depersonalization manifesting as cynicism, is likely to exponentially exacerbate such tensions and impede attempts to improve organizational culture.

Difficult or disruptive behavior can have a significant damaging effect on organizational culture. According to Karen Weiner, MD, MMM, chief medical officer at Oregon Medical Group in Eugene, Oregon, such behavior on the part of physicians is almost always due to their perception that their ability to provide quality care is being compromised: "Inappropriate responses or angry yelling happens because the physician felt unable to provide the quality of care he or she wanted. That's an important value that the majority of physicians share...If an organizational leader has a lot of dissatisfied physicians, what that's telling you is your physicians are perceiving barriers to providing quality care. It's a strong indicator that something's wrong." Rather than being a separate and distinct problem, disruptive behavior is a signal that underlying quality issues exist.

Burnout and its underlying drivers (described in Part 2) hinder an organization's capacity to recruit and retain talented physicians and other staff. Research has shown that burnout correlates with intention to leave. (Shanafelt 2009 archives; Rabatin 2016) As Maslach has described it, "[Burnout is] a key factor in low worker morale, absenteeism, and high job turnover, for a common response to burnout is to quit and get out." (Maslach 1976) Higher turnover places additional stress on the remaining clinicians, increasing their risk of burnout.

Gifted clinicians want to work in positive environments with great outcomes. They are less likely to stay in organizations with low morale and widespread burnout.

## Financial performance

Physician burnout also exacts a significant toll on an organization's finances, including additional costs and lost revenue. Burnout costs money. It is associated with an increased risk of medical errors and negative effects on the patient-physician relationship, which may result in more malpractice claims. The propensity of physicians with burnout to leave practice also has direct financial consequences. The cost of recruiting one primary care physician in 1999 was estimated to be $250,000.

(Buchbinder 1999) A 2004 study estimated the lost revenue from turnover to be about $2 million. (Misra-Hebert 2004) These costs are considered to be far greater today. Many health care leaders with whom we have spoken estimated the cost of replacing a primary care physician to be $400,000 or more. A recent study in Canada estimated that the national cost of burnout was $213.1 million annually, with $185.2 million of that due to early retirement and $27.9 million due to reduced clinical hours. (Dewa 2014) Published studies of the current costs of recruitment and replacement in the United States are lacking.

Beyond the malpractice-related and recruitment costs, burned-out physicians are simply less productive than their counterparts without burnout. A 2001 study documented that burnout is associated with lower workplace productivity and efficiency. (Linzer 2001) Burnout among physicians is also predictive of reduced work output. Tait Shanafelt and his colleagues at the Mayo Clinic have documented that physicians with burnout symptoms were significantly more likely to reduce their work hours (that is, full-time equivalents [FTEs]) over the subsequent two years, as measured by payroll records. (Shanafelt 2016) A national study of physicians found that 44 percent of the more than 20,000 physicians who responded were planning to take steps that would result in reduced patient access to their services, including retiring, shifting to part-time hours, leaving practice, reducing the number of patients seen, or closing their practice to new patients. The study authors estimated that these changes could result in the loss of tens of thousands of physician FTEs when extrapolated to the entire physician workforce. (The Physicians Foundation 2014)

How much revenue are we talking about? According to some estimates, a primary care physician directs about $1.6 million per year to his or her health care organization through referrals, imaging, and procedures. (Merritt Hawkins 2013) A 10 percent reduction in FTEs due to burnout represents a loss of $160,000 for each physician who cuts back on patient care time.

In addition, when physicians cut back or leave practice, their patients may choose to affiliate with another organization, representing a lost revenue stream. Whether these patients choose to go or stay, they risk disruptions to care continuity. As stated in a recent *Health Affairs* post,

"Lost productivity for physicians, nurses, and other members of the health care team contribute[s] to additional costs, and associated attrition leads to loss of continuity across the care team and care settings." (Shin 2016)

## Overall performance and organizational resilience

Burnout endangers an organization's ability to reach its strategic goals. Physicians who are burned out or dissatisfied are less likely to have the will to collaborate or the interest in collaborating with the administration to achieve organizational goals. They are less likely to be fully engaged and involved, to champion improvement efforts and embrace the many challenging changes related to health reform. Weiner told us that reducing burnout among the physicians in the multispecialty group was a top priority. "When I joined the board and saw what we were trying to do, I realized that burnout was preventing us from reaching our goals. We had to take steps to address it or we couldn't move forward." Indeed, the creators of the term "Quadruple Aim" coined the term after touring physician practices across the United States and hearing a common refrain: "We have adopted the Triple Aim as our framework, but the stressful work life of our clinicians and staff impacts our ability to achieve the three aims." (Bodenheimer 2014) The authors proposed adding a fourth aim: improving the work life of health care clinicians and staff.

As mentioned previously, organizational leaders would do well to take physician burnout seriously for another reason: physician distress, burnout, and disruptive behavior reflect as other problems, such as communication gaps, inefficient workplace practices, and safety issues, that adversely affect patient care and organizational performance.

Physician burnout also endangers an organization's ability to be nimble when facing environmental change. To be successful in today's market, health care organizations need a critical mass of talented, engaged, and energized professionals who will all pull in the same direction. Only with engaged physicians on board will leaders be able to implement new strategies effectively to deal quickly with a new external pressure or to capitalize on a new growth opportunity.

## THE EFFECTS OF BURNOUT ON THE HEALTH CARE SYSTEM

The effect of physician burnout on the larger health care system is beyond the scope of this book. However, we would be remiss if we failed to point out that employers, public and commercial health care payers, and society at large stand to be markedly affected by the growing tide of physician dissatisfaction and burnout. As Maslach wrote, "There is little doubt that burnout plays a major role in the poor delivery of health and welfare services to people in need of them. They wait longer to receive less attention and less care." (Maslach 1976) With physician burnout continuing in its present state, patients will suffer from reduced care practices, an increased risk of medical errors, strained relationships with their physicians, and greater restrictions in their access to care. Employers and payers will bear the brunt of additional costs and floundering improvement initiatives. Society will struggle with additional costs and a worsening of the projected physician shortage.

As F. Joseph Lee, MD, and his colleagues stated in a 2008 article, "If fewer physicians choose to practice family medicine, this will aggravate the existing shortage of family physicians and further reduce access to primary care." (Lee 2008) Given that training a new physician is a decade-long process, the loss of midcareer, seasoned professionals from health care is a cost none of us can afford to ignore.

*♫♫*

To effectively prevent the consequences of physician burnout, we need to understand and address its root causes. In Part 2 we will consider the underlying factors that are causing such widespread distress among physicians.

## REFERENCES

Ariely D, Lanier WL. Disturbing trends in physician burnout and satisfaction with work-life balance: dealing with malady among the nation's healers. *Mayo Clin Proc.* 2015 Dec;90(12):1593–1596.

Bodenheimer T, Sinsky C. From triple to quadruple aim: care of the patient requires care of the provider. *Ann Fam Med.* 2014;12(6):573–576.

Buchbinder SB, Wilson M, Melick CF, Powe NR. Estimates of costs of primary care physician turnover. *Am J Manag Care.* 1999;5(11):1431–1438.

Dewa CS, Jacobs P, Thanh NX, Loong D. An estimate of the cost of burnout on early retirement and reduction in clinical hours of practicing physicians in Canada. *BMC Health Services Research.* 2014;14:254.

Dyrbye LN, Massie FS, Eacker A, et al. Relationship between burnout and professional conduct and attitudes among US medical students. *JAMA.* 2010;304(11):1173–1180.

Dyrbye LN, Thomas MR, Massie FS, et al. Burnout and suicidal ideation among US medical students. *Ann Intern Med.* 2008;149(5):334–341.

DeVoe J, Fryer Jr GE, Hargraves JL, Phillips RL, Green LA. Does career dissatisfaction affect the ability of family physicians to deliver high-quality patient care? *J Fam Pract.* 2002;51(3):223–228.

DeVoe J, Fryer GE Jr, Straub A, McCann J, Fairbrother G. Congruent satisfaction: is there geographic correlation between patient and physician satisfaction? *Med Care.* 2007;45(1):88–94.

Fahrenkopf AM, Sectish TC, Barger LK, et al. Rates of medication errors among depressed and burnt-out residents: prospective cohort study. *BMJ.* 2008;336(7642):488–491.

Firth-Cozens J, Greenhalgh J. Doctors' perceptions of the links between stress and lowered clinical care. *Soc Sci Med.* 1997;44(7):1017–1022.

Gold KJ, Sen A, Schwenk TL. Details on suicide among US physicians: data from the National Violent Death Reporting System. *Gen Hosp Psychiatry.* 2013;35(1):45–49.

Golkar A, Johansson E, Kasahara M, Osika W, Perski A, Savic I. The influence of work-related chronic stress on the regulation of emotion and on functional connectivity in the brain. *PLoS One.* 2014;9(9):e104550.

Grundy P. Primary partner care. 2016. Available at: http://primarypartnercare.com/about. Accessed September 9, 2016.

Haas JS, Cook EF, Puopolo AL, Burstin HR, Cleary PD, Brennan TA. Is the professional satisfaction of general internists associated with patient satisfaction? *J Gen Intern Med.* 2000;15(2):122–128.

Hemp P. Presenteeism: at work—but out of it. *Harv Bus Rev.* October 2004.

Iannelli RJ, Finlayson AJ, Brown KP, et al. Suicidal behavior among physicians referred for fitness-for-duty evaluation. *Gen Hosp Psychiatry.* 2014;36(6):732–736.

Landon BE, Reschovsky J, Blumenthal D. Changes in career satisfaction among primary care and specialist physicians, 1997–2001. *JAMA.* 2003;289(4):442–449.

Lee FJ, Stewart M, Brown JB. Stress, burnout, and strategies for reducing them: what's the situation among Canadian family physicians? *Can Fam Physician.* 2008;54(2):234–235.

Linzer M, Manwell LB, Williams ES, et al. Working conditions in primary care: physician reactions and care quality. *Ann Intern Med.* 2009;151(1):28–36.

Linzer M, Visser MR, Oort FJ, Smets EM, McMurray JE, de Haes HC. Predicting and preventing physician burnout: results from the United States and the Netherlands. *Am J Med.* 2001;111(2):170–175.

Mani A, Mullainathan S, Shafir E, Zhao J. Poverty impedes cognitive function. *Science.* 2013;341(6149):976–980.

Maslach C. Burned-out. *Hum Behav* 1976;9:16–22.

Merritt Hawkins. 2013 Physician inpatient/outpatient revenue survey. 2013. Available at: http://www.merritthawkins.com/uploadedFiles/MerrittHawkins/Pdf/mha2013revenuesurveyPDF.pdf. Accessed June 26, 2016.

Misra-Hebert AD, Kay R, Stoller JK. A review of physician turnover: rates, causes, and consequences. *Am J Med Qual.* 2004;19(2):56–66.

Oreskovich MR, Kaups KL, Balch CM, et al. Prevalence of alcohol use disorders among American surgeons. *Arch Surg.* 2012;147(2):168–174.

The Physicians Foundation. 2014 survey of America's physicians: practice, patterns, and perspective. 2014. Available at: http://www.physiciansfoundation.org/uploads/default/2014_Physicians_Foundation_Biennial_Physician_Survey_Report.pdf. Accessed April 29, 2016.

Press Ganey. Every voice matters: the bottom line on employee and physician engagement. 2015. Available at: http://www.pressganey.com/resources/white-papers/every-voice-matters-the-bottom-line-on-employee-physician-engagement. Accessed October 27, 2016.

Rabatin J, Williams E, Baier Manwell L, Schwartz MD, Brown RL, Linzer M. Predictors and outcomes of burnout in primary care physicians. *J Prim Care Community Health.* 2016;7(1):41–43.

Schernhammer ES, Colditz GA. Suicide rates among physicians: a quantitative and gender assessment (meta-analysis). *Am J Psychiatry.* 2004 Dec;161(12):2295–2302.

Shanafelt TD, Balch CM, Bechamps G, et al. Burnout and medical errors among American surgeons. *Ann Surg.* 2010;251(6):995–1000.

Shanafelt TD, Bradley KA, Wipf JE, Back AL. Burnout and self-reported patient care in an internal medicine residency program. *Ann Intern Med.* 2002;136(5):358–367.

Shanafelt TD, Mungo M, Schmitgen J, et al. Longitudinal study evaluating the association between physician burnout and changes in professional work effort. *Mayo Clin Proc.* 2016;91(4):422–431.

Shanafelt TD, West CP, Sloan JA, et al. Career fit and burnout among academic faculty. *Arch Intern Med.* 2009;169(10):990–995.

Shin A, Gandhi T, Herzig S. Make the clinician burnout epidemic a national priority. 2016. Available at: http://healthaffairs.org/blog/2016/04/21/make-the-clinician-burnout-epidemic-a-national-priority. Accessed April 29, 2016.

Torre DM, Wang NY, Meoni LA, Young JH, Klag MJ, Ford DE. Suicide compared to other causes of mortality in physicians. *Suicide Life Threat Behav.* 2005;35(2):146–153.

Wallace JE, Lemaire JB, Ghali WA. Physician wellness: a missing quality indicator. *Lancet.* 2009;374:1714–1721.

West CP, Huschka MM, Novotny PJ, et al. Association of perceived medical errors with resident distress and empathy: a prospective longitudinal study. *JAMA.* 2006;296(9):1071–1078.

West CP, Tan AD, Shanafelt TD. Association of resident fatigue and distress with occupational blood and body fluid exposures and motor vehicle incidents. *Mayo Clin Proc.* 2012;87(12):1138–1144.

Williams ES, Manwell LB, Konrad TR, Linzer M. The relationship of organizational culture, stress, satisfaction, and burnout with physician-reported error and suboptimal patient care: results from the MEMO study. *Health Care Manage Rev.* 2007;32(3):203–212.

# PART 2

## IDENTIFYING THE DRIVERS OF BURNOUT

P hysician burnout is multifactorial. There is no single explanation for burnout in an individual physician or for the drastic uptick across all specialties in recent years. Understanding the variety of factors that are responsible for physician burnout will help highlight key leverage points for prevention.

Health care leaders may believe they are already aware of the factors that explain the burnout epidemic: for example, new external mandates, changes related to health reform, and physician resistance to new practice realities and team-based care. Physicians may believe burnout is caused by frustrations such as the adaptation needed for electronic health records, increased productivity demands, and the reduction in direct patient care time. Although all of these factors can increase the risk of burnout, other, less obvious, factors are important as well. Part 2 will cover both the obvious and less obvious causes of burnout.

We have developed a visual model (figure 2) that illustrates our thinking about the root causes of burnout.

In this model, physicians are placed in the center circle. Physicians bring to their practice individual liabilities and strengths, which can make them more or less susceptible to stress. The next ring in the model represents drivers in the workplace environment. These factors, such as inefficient patient care processes, exert pressure on physicians and sap their resilience in the face of stressors. The outermost ring in the model represents the drivers external to the health care organization, such as new reimbursement penalties, that exert pressure on the workplace and,

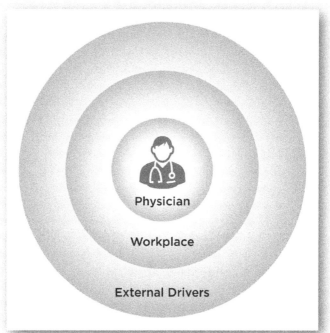

Figure 2: Visual Model of the Root Causes of Physician Burnout

in turn, on physicians. In our model, the demands from the external environment, the immediate practice setting, and any personal factors within the physician can overwhelm the resilience of the physician to stress, resulting in burnout.

In the current health care environment, the external demands are heightened by new expectations regarding patient satisfaction scores, quality metrics, and productivity, while the capacity of physicians is reduced by factors such as greater time demands of data entry and coding requirements. The result? An ever-tightening vise, with the factors in the outermost ring exerting pressure on the middle ring, which, in turn, squeezes physicians and other care providers.

In the next chapter, we will consider the factors intrinsic to physicians that may increase their susceptibility to developing burnout when exposed to work situations with high levels of chronic stress.

# CHAPTER 3

## PHYSICIAN FACTORS

*The profession has changed around us, yet our macho culture and industrialized work environment have failed to accommodate to the reality of this occupational health crisis and the burnout it is producing.*
—STEVE ADELMAN, MD, DIRECTOR OF PHYSICIAN HEALTH SERVICES AT THE MASSACHUSETTS MEDICAL SOCIETY[1]

*I feel this enormous responsibility. I keep waking up in the middle of the night, knowing that things fall through the cracks. It's exhausting, and it never ends. I just wish I had a quick exit plan.*
—MIDCAREER CARDIOLOGIST WITH BURNOUT

Physician-related factors that can increase the risk of burnout fall into five categories: stresses inherent to the practice of medicine, common traits and characteristics of physicians, mental health of physicians, prevailing culture in medical training and the profession at large, and other individual factors.

---

1 Adelman S. It's getting hot in here: the latest on physician burnout. *Vital Signs.* [Newsletter]. Massachusetts Medical Society. March 2016. Available at: http://www.massmed.org/news-and-publications/vital-signs/vital-signs-march-2016-%28pdf%29. Accessed May 7, 2016.

## THE INHERENT STRESSES OF MEDICAL PRACTICE

The vast majority of physicians enter the profession of medicine because of an altruistic desire to alleviate suffering. Many feel called to the profession with a willingness to make personal sacrifices to benefit others. Although many other professions share this attribute, medicine is somewhat unique in the long period of required training, the intensely emotional aspects of the work, and the level of dedication required to pursue the profession. Other fields may involve more risk or a similar degree of stress, but the practice of medicine carries with it certain unique stresses.

Arguably the most powerful of these stresses is that of feeling responsible for other people's lives. Most physicians find ways to cope with this aspect of medicine. Others find the responsibility overwhelming, substantially increasing their susceptibility to adverse responses if they cannot find a healthy, effective way to handle it. As one physician who left midway through radiology training stated in an interview, "I never found a way to cope with the sense of responsibility. I liked the technical and intellectual aspects of radiology, but that sense of responsibility is a little thing that is actually *very* big. The number one cause of burnout in my case was the underlying anxiety that a mistake would harm others." In addition to the anxiety about making a mistake and the gravity of being responsible for other's lives, physicians face the stress of potential malpractice claims. Being named in a suit, whether it is dropped, settled out of court, or brought to trial, is one of the most stressful events in a physician's life. (Sanbar 2007)

Physicians face stressful practice situations on a daily basis: a patient's unexpected death, the loss of a newborn, an angry patient, giving bad news, or apologizing for an error. They may struggle to find places where they feel comfortable talking about the emotional toll of these experiences. They may fear appearing weak or unprofessional. As Paul Melinkovich, MD, president of the Colorado Medical Services Board and director of Community Health Services at Denver Health, described his experience at the safety net hospital, "It's a leap to accept that you cannot save all your patients, and you must just be there and offer help. There are a lot of factors in their environment and social situation totally outside our influence that make it hard for them to do things that would improve their life. It's hard to see that day after day. It helps if you're on a supportive team, so you can talk it through."

Another inherent stress of medicine is the associated time demands. The long, time-intensive hours spent in training mean that many physicians delay personal milestones, such as marriage and childbearing. Once in practice, the average physician works more hours than his or her professional colleagues (50 hours versus 40), with four out of ten physicians working 60 hours or more per week. (Shanafelt 2015) Time demands can reduce a physician's ability to bounce back after a particularly long or exhausting day. In addition, the long hours and the often inflexible schedule can take a toll on a physician's life outside of work. Physician coach Michelle Mudge-Riley sees work-life conflict in most of her clients, although the source of the conflict tends to differ by gender. "Women feel more guilty about home and family and keeping up with responsibilities there. Men feel the responsibility of being good breadwinners."

In an interview, George Palma, MD, medical director at Simpler and former assistant physician-in-chief at Kaiser Permanente, recalled the stress of balancing home and work responsibilities, saying, "In my private practice before joining a large medical group, I was on call every fourth night, which was doable until we had children. Eventually I found myself resenting call and the demands of patients, because I felt I had no time to be a person." A physician who left practice because of burnout described the conflict she experienced when doing the "extra" work that was important for providing compassionate care: "If I stayed for a one-hour family conference, which was uncompensated time, I would end up leaving several hours late. But I felt it necessary to practice humane medicine. Once I was a mother, I realized I could not make it work and be the kind of mom I wanted to be. The job proved unsustainable for me."

## COMMON TRAITS AND CHARACTERISTICS OF PHYSICIANS

On the whole, physicians share certain traits and characteristics. One researcher summed up one common trait by saying, "There is no doubt that compulsiveness is the hallmark of the physician's personality." (Gabbard 1985) The compulsiveness can present as difficulty relaxing, reluctance to take vacations, an excessive sense of responsibility for things outside of one's control, guilt, and doubt. (Gabbard 1985)

In our experience as physicians, our "tribe" tends to be perfectionistic, conscientious, self-critical, and independent. We generally like to be autonomous, and we value our independence.

The fact that physicians tend to display these traits is not surprising. It makes sense that people who are drawn to the profession would share certain characteristics, such as intellectual curiosity and a desire to help others. Similarly, individuals with a certain level of mental aptitude and certain personality traits are more likely to successfully navigate the rigors of pre-medical studies, medical school admission and completion, and residency training. The first hurdle to becoming a physician, pre-medical studies, emphasizes traits of competitiveness with classmates, favors individual success over team success, and selects for an ability to perform well on standardized tests.

Not only does the selection and training process favor some traits that may be antithetical to the characteristics that society most values in physicians, such as empathy and the ability to work well in teams, it also favors some traits that might increase the risk of burnout under chronic stress or after training is complete. For example, a professionally desirable trait like conscientiousness can become a liability in a physician driven to complete every task to perfection by him- or herself, because he or she will experience time pressure when new performance expectations or difficulties with technology result in additional work demands. Paul Grundy of IBM explained it to us this way: "It's not possible for physicians to keep up with the pace and changes in medicine. Trying to keep all the information in their heads while working at the center of the process, physicians run into cognitive breakdown."

Given the possibility that certain traits might increase the susceptibility to burnout, one might consider screening for them at medical school admission. However, this is not an effective strategy for building a population of talented, empathetic, mission-driven physicians. In fact, according to Tait Shanafelt of the Mayo Clinic, research suggests that individuals who are more callous and less empathetic may be at lower risk for burnout. (Medscape article) In a 2012 keynote address at the International Conference on Physician Health, he opined that the physicians who may appear to be less prone to burnout may also be the physicians least committed to their work. (Collier 2012) In trying to pre-select such physicians, "You would weed out the very people you would want to be your colleagues," he concluded.

## THE MENTAL HEALTH OF PHYSICIANS

Physicians suffer from certain mental health conditions at rates that are as high as or higher than those of the general population. The incidence of depression in medical students and residents is in the range of 15 to 30 percent, which is higher than in the general population. (Zoccolillo 1986; Givens 2002; Shanafelt 2002; Fahrenkopf 2008) When training is completed, these rates decline to rates similar to those of the general population, about 13 percent for male physicians and 20 percent for female physicians. (Frank 1999) Studies have shown, however, that certain personality traits that are common among physicians, such as perfectionism, may increase an individual's risk for depression and substance abuse. (Vaillant 1972) And, as mentioned in Chapter 2, physicians are at much greater risk of suicide than are other professionals or the general population. (Schermhammer 2004)

The fact that physicians are susceptible to certain mental health conditions might not be an issue at all, except that for a number of reasons, these conditions are often untreated, or insufficiently treated, in physicians. Physicians often avoid revealing a problem, or they self-prescribe. (Watts 2005; Baldwin 1997) A study of physicians and dentists who sought help for substance abuse or a mental health condition found a high level of severity, suggesting that they had delayed seeking treatment. (Brooks 2011) Physicians often fear the loss of their license or privileges if they reveal the presence of a mental health condition. Current regulations in many states and many organizational policies require such disclosure. One researcher put it this way: "Unfortunately, the culture of medicine usually accords a low priority to physician mental health despite evidence of a high rate of untreated mood disorders and an increased burden of suicide. Too often, depression remains unrecognized or untreated until a physician's personal distress compromises his or her capacity to care for patients. For physicians seeking help, there is often a punitive response, including discrimination in medical licensing, hospital privileges, and professional advancement." (Balsch 2009)

When untreated, mental health conditions, such as depression and bipolar disorder, can adversely affect physicians' resilience to stressful work environments and potentially in their ability to perform effectively.

## THE CULTURE IN TRAINING AND THE MEDICAL PROFESSION

Culture has been defined as "integrated patterns of human behavior that include the language, thoughts, communications, actions, customs, beliefs, values, and institutions of racial, ethnic, religious, or social groups." (Office of Minority Health, 2002) It involves thoughts and beliefs about group norms, and it shapes what individuals in a group believe and how they behave. The culture in which physicians train and practice affects them; it creates unspoken expectations about their work, how they spend their time, how they view themselves, and how they treat colleagues, other staff, and patients.

The prevailing culture in medicine may reinforce beliefs that can make physicians both more effective at their work and at greater risk for burnout. Gwen Adshead, professor of psychiatry at Gresham College in the United Kingdom, and her colleagues have pointed out that the medical culture may support and select for the following beliefs: (Adshead 2010)

- Narcissism: I am the greatest.
- Perfectionism: I must do this right, and mistakes are intolerable in me/others.
- Compulsiveness: I have to do this, and I can't give up till I finish.
- Denigration of vulnerability: People who need help are failures.
- Shame: If I am in need, I am a failure.

Physicians are strongly affected by the culture in which they practice, beginning with acculturation during training.

## TRAINING ACCULTURATION

When future physicians enter medical school, they learn about their new profession through formal lessons and through the unspoken "hidden curriculum." As one author describes it, "Although it is not a part of the formal curriculum, the hidden curriculum often dictates certain customs, rituals, and rules of conduct thereby, defining the cultural milieu of medicine."(Boutin-Foster 2008) The hidden curriculum may undermine what is learned in the classroom. According to Anthony Montgomery, PhD, associate professor of the psychology of work and organizations at the University of Macedonia in Greece, a classic example of the hidden curriculum at work is attending physicians failing to treat patients with respect. "Patient neglect, that is, legally doing your job but not really doing it, also reflects the hidden curriculum," he told us.

The hidden curriculum also teaches trainees what is expected of them as professionals. Often the message is to ignore their physical and emotional needs. One physician we interviewed shared a legend passed from resident to resident during her training that exemplifies the hero aspect of medical culture. "A pregnant female surgeon self-inserted a Foley catheter in preparation for a Whipple procedure. After completing the closure some eight hours later, the surgeon walked over to the maternity unit and gave birth. Whether the story was true or not almost didn't matter. It was perpetuated for a reason. It told us what it takes to be successful and that you better not complain if you're tired or hungry."

Another lesson that physicians learn through the hidden curriculum is how individuals with a higher standing in a power dynamic behave toward those with a lower standing. A 2011 survey found that more than 80 percent of medical students had been publicly humiliated or belittled in the course of their training and that 18 percent had been asked to perform personal tasks for an instructor. (Mavis 2014) Montgomery and others have labeled such behavior bullying. "It's a basic psychology premise that those who are bullied will bully others. People treat others with the same behavior they see modeled," he said in an interview. Perhaps this unspoken lesson explains the documented loss of empathy that occurs during training. Research has shown that interns display progressively less empathy over the course of the internship year. (Bellini 2002) This drop occurs despite the fact that they are more empathetic on average than comparison groups when they begin training.

As one physician described in an online post on KevinMD, "Many of [the residents] match in our residency program with their wellness accounts already in negative balance, or precariously close to empty—the product of an obsolete, hierarchical medical education system that still often relies on overwork and humiliation as a sort of rite of passage with no formal teaching on how to deal with emotions, time management, financial or business competence, or self-care." (Gallardo 2016)

Data that Montgomery and his team collected from nine countries indicate that bullying behavior during training may be escalating (personal communication, December 18, 2015): "The selection process to enter medical school in some countries is increasingly competitive. The process tends to select individuals who are strong scholars but may be weaker in the 'soft' skills, such as communication and empathy. Plus, the competitive environment makes it difficult for trainees to take a team focus."

The taxing schedule and time demands of clinical training have been a national focus in recent years; regulations in the United States now restrict the number of hours that residents can work and stipulate hours off for sleep. However, these regulations may not be sufficient to create a culture that fosters resiliency rather than burnout. As Ted Hamilton, MD, MBA, vice president for medical mission at Adventist Health System and chair of the executive committee of the Coalition for Physician Well-Being, said in an interview, "The work culture for physicians has been crushing for a long time…We applaud the new regulations for humanizing residency, with no more than an 80-hour work week, no more than every third night on call, and at least one day off per week. *What* are we thinking? When human beings get tired, they don't give the care that any of us would want for ourselves." For some trainees, the culture and experience are simply unendurable. As a resident who left training midway through told us, "Eventually I thought, 'No one forced me to be a physician. I can get out. Life doesn't have to be this bad.'"

## THE CULTURE OF MEDICINE

The culture of the profession of medicine does little to encourage self-care or a healthy work-life balance. Rather, it creates the expectation that the norm is long work days, insufficient time off to re-energize, and little opportunity for personal activities. This aspect of the culture of medicine, when combined with the personality trait of compulsiveness, may reduce the likelihood that physicians will prioritize stress reduction techniques, such as meditation and mindfulness.

Within this culture, physicians learn that it is best to hide any weaknesses. As Mudge-Riley told us, "Burnout still carries a stigma. We don't want to say we don't know anything, let alone admit when we're in trouble." The resident mentioned at the end of the "Training Acculturation" section described his experience with this aspect of medical culture, saying, "I did not go to anyone to talk about the emotional stress I was feeling. I felt I needed to be 'professional.' I wanted to project the right demeanor, like I have it all together. I didn't want to appear weak or unreliable…until the end when hiding it was not an option."

The unspoken expectation to be superhuman and to ignore or suppress emotional and physical needs can be harmful to physicians in several ways. They may neglect basic self-care, setting them up for later impairment. They may also struggle to deal effectively with emotionally laden experiences involving patients and families.

According to James Hereford, chief operating officer at Stanford University Medical Center, burnout is not surprising, given the current culture in medicine. "The training says to be a hero and that you are ultimately responsible for everything. But we have not had a system that helps clinicians by making the right thing the easy thing to do. No wonder there is burnout. It's amazing, given the system, that it's not worse."

The combination of a superhuman mentality, which many physicians adopt in training, and a workplace that involves increasing stresses and demands is a recipe for work-life imbalance and burnout. Physicians caught in this dynamic feel the imperative to do "whatever it takes" for optimal patient care in circumstances in which achieving that is impossible. National studies by the Mayo Clinic show that physicians are increasingly experiencing worse work-life balance (even compared with other professionals) and more burnout. (Shanafelt 2015)

Lesley Doherty, RN, the former CEO of Bolton NHS Foundation Trust in the United Kingdom, described the other side of this challenge to us. As training hours have decreased, physicians in training are increasingly stressed by their lack of clinical skills. Lack of confidence is becoming a stressor for physicians and the nurses with whom they work.

## OTHER INDIVIDUAL FACTORS

In addition to the four factors discussed so far, several other individual factors can influence a physician's resilience to stress and burnout. A primary stressor for many residents and early-career physicians today is debt. According to the American Association of Medical Colleges, more than 80 percent of medical school graduates carry educational debt, with an average amount of almost $180,000. About 1 in 10 graduates owes more than $300,000. (AAMC 2015)

In addition, unfulfilled expectations may affect a physician's experience of medical practice. Trainees may look toward the end of their residency and fellowship years with an expectation of substantial improvement in their life situation. For some, however, this is not the case. A hospitalist who left practice early in her career told us, "I thought when my residency was ending that there was a light at the end of the tunnel. So, I kept going and going. And then I realized it was a train." She told us that while training felt like a collective effort, practice was isolating and associated with greater productivity demands. "In residency, there was a sense of camaraderie and teamwork. We were fighting a good fight, even if at 4:00 a.m. In private practice, I felt like I was trying to fight the good fight by myself with no one else around. Seeing how different and isolating it was felt like a big blow."

Given the recent trends in physician employment and additional external mandates, many physicians may feel dissatisfied with the low degree of independence they find in current practice. Individuals drawn to the practice of medicine tend to desire autonomy. Mudge-Riley sees this in her clients. "Physicians come to the profession because they want to feel empowered. Sometimes this can lead to stress when they are asked to standardize practices. They can feel less empowered." Physicians who especially value autonomy may be experiencing more stress and frustration with recent changes in the external environment that are affecting their practice experience.

*∬∬*

It may be easier—or perhaps human nature—to identify physician burnout as caused by individual weakness or a certain susceptibility. Rather than searching out systems issues, it may be tempting to think of the inherent stresses of practice, the traits and characteristics of physicians, mental health issues, and the effects of the culture of medicine as being the culprits. However, the widespread nature of burnout today indicates that clinicians with burnout are not weak links but rather canaries in the coal mine.

As Tait Shanafelt of the Mayo Clinic and his co-authors commented in their 2012 study, "The fact that almost 1 in 2 US physicians has symptoms of burnout implies that the origins of this problem are rooted in the environment and care delivery system rather than in the personal characteristics of a few susceptible individuals." (Shanafelt 2012)

We 'll discuss the workplace drivers responsible for burnout in more detail in the next chapter.

## REFERENCES

Adshead G. Disruptive and distressed doctors: relevance of personality disorder. [Slide presentation]. December 2010. European Association for Physician Health. 2nd Annual Conference. Barcelona, Spain. Available at: http://www.eaph.eu/pdf/Disruptive+and+distressed+doctors+-+Relevance+of+personality+disorder.pdf. Accessed May 7, 2016.

American Association of Medical Colleges. Medical student education: debt, costs, and loan repayment fact card. October 2015. Available at: https://www.aamc.org/download/447254/data/debtfactcard.pdf. Accessed May 5, 2016.

Balch CM, Freischlag JA, Shanafelt TD. Stress and burnout among surgeons: understanding and managing the syndrome and avoiding the adverse consequences. *Arch Surg.* 2009;144(4):371–376.

Baldwin PJ, Dodd M, Wrate RM. Young doctors' health—II. Health and health behaviour. *Soc Sci Med.* 1997;45(1):41–44.

Bellini LM, Baime M, Shea JA. Variation of mood and empathy during internship. *JAMA.* 2002;287(23):3143–3146.

Boutin-Foster C, Foster JC, Konopasek L. Viewpoint: physician, know thyself: the professional culture of medicine as a framework for teaching cultural competence. *Acad Med.* 2008;83(1):106–111.

Brooks SK, Chalder T, Gerada C. Doctors vulnerable to psychological distress and addictions: treatment from the Practitioner Health Programme. *J Ment Health.* 2011;20(2):157–164.

Collier R. The "physician personality" and other factors in physician health. *CMAJ.* 2012;184(18):1980.

Fahrenkopf AM, Sectish TC, Barger LK, et al. Rates of medication errors among depressed and burnt-out residents: prospective cohort study. *BMJ.* 2008;336(7642):488–491.

Frank E, Dingle AD. Self-reported depression and suicide attempts among US women physicians. *Am J Psychiatry.* 1999;156:1887–1894.

Gabbard GO. The role of compulsiveness in the normal physician. *JAMA.* 1985;254(20):2926–2929.

Gallardo S. A Generation-X physician embraces the millennial doctor perspective. [Internet]. February 21, 2016. KevinMD.com. Available at: http://www.kevinmd.com/blog/2016/02/generation-x-physician-embraces-millennial-doctor-perspective.html.

Givens JL, Tjia J. Depressed medical students' use of mental health services and barriers to use. *Acad Med.* 2002;77(9):918–921.

Mavis B, Sousa A, Lipscomb W, Rappley MD. Learning about medical student mistreatment from responses to the medical school graduation questionnaire. *Acad Med.* 2014;89(5):705–711.

Office of Minority Health, US Department of Health and Human Services. *Teaching Cultural Competence in Health Care: A Review of Current Concepts, Policies, and Practices.* Washington, DC: US Department of Health and Human Services. 2002.

Sanbar SS, Firestone MH. Medical malpractice stress syndrome. In: American College of Legal Medicine. *The Medical Malpractice Survival Handbook.* Philadelphia: Mosby Inc. 2007.

Schernhammer ES, Colditz GA. Suicide rates among physicians: a quantitative and gender assessment (meta-analysis). *Am J Psychiatry.* 2004 Dec;161(12):2295–2302.

Scutter L, Shanafelt T. Two sides of the physician coin: burnout and well-being. [Internet]. February 9, 2015. Medscape. Available at: http://www.medscape.com/viewarticle/839439. Accessed May 7, 2016.

Shanafelt TD, Hasan O, Dyrbye LN, et al. Changes in burnout and satisfaction with work-life balance in physicians and the general

US working population between 2011 and 2014. *Mayo Clin Proc.* 2015;90(12):1600–1613.

Shanafelt TD, Boone S, Tan L, et al. Burnout and satisfaction with work-life balance among US physicians relative to the general US population. *Arch Intern Med.* 2012;172:1377–1385.

Shanafelt TD, Bradley KA, Wipf JE, Back AL. Burnout and self-reported patient care in an internal medicine residency program. *Ann Intern Med.* 2002;136(5):358–367.

Vaillant GE, Sobowale NC, McArthur C. Some psychological vulnerabilities of physicians. *N Engl J Med.* 1972;287:372–375.

Watts, G. Doctors, drink and drugs. *BMJ Careers.* 2005;331:105–106.

Zoccolillo M, Murphy GE, Wetzel RD. Depression among medical students. *J Affect Disord.* 1986;11(1):91–96.

# CHAPTER 4

## Workplace Drivers of Burnout in the General Population

> *We create stressful work situations and then try to treat people, but we don't go to the root cause.*
> —Bob Chapman, author of *Everybody Matters: The Extraordinary Power of Caring for Your People Like Family*, personal communication, December 17, 2015

> *One of the biggest challenges is that people tend to think of burnout in terms of individual factors and individual responsibility. They tend to blame the individual. Despite research that shows the importance of the environment, background, and situation, people still think, "Too bad that person can't handle it." A harder message to hear, or a more overwhelming one, is that the problem is more than the individual.*
> —Christina Maslach, PhD, professor emeritus in the Department of Psychology at the University of California, Berkeley, personal communication, February 1, 2016

Physician burnout differs from burnout in the general population because physicians are subject not only to all the worker-workplace mismatches that drive burnout in the general population, but also to additional factors that are unique to their role as physicians. In this chapter we'll discuss the workplace drivers of burnout that researchers have identified for the general population and relate the data to physicians' experience. In the next chapter we'll cover the workplace drivers that other researchers have identified as specific to physicians.

Clearly, burnout is not caused by a single issue; it is multifactorial. We firmly believe, however, that a substantial portion of the risk stems from factors in the workplace. Research supports this premise. A 2015 study of primary care physicians identified various workplace factors as being highly predictive of burnout. (Gregory 2015) Chief among these were physician workload, degree of physician control, and congruence between the physician's values and those of the administration. Mark Linzer of Hennepin County Medical Center has estimated that practice factors predict about 50 percent of the risk of burnout (personal communication, June 27, 2016).

In an interview, Wayne Sotile of the Center for Physician Resilience compared the current situation in health care to a five-way intersection with physicians standing at the crossroads and no one directing traffic. He said, "It is as if we are asking physicians, 'Please stop bleeding,' instead of installing a traffic signal to fix the problem." His statement is especially striking, because his work focuses on improving the resilience of individual physicians to the effects of stress. The fact that burnout affects more than half of physicians today suggests the presence of drivers outside the individual. What has changed in the environment in which physicians practice that explains this massive uptick in burnout?

## A CHANGING WORKPLACE

Anyone who has seen Robert Young playing Marcus Welby, M.D. on the old television series may yearn for that nostalgic era, when a dedicated primary care doctor ran his own office and seemed to have an abundance of time for addressing his patients' medical and psychosocial needs, both in the office and in the hospital. As patients, we yearn to have a physician who will care for us with this level of personal attention. As physicians, we wish we could work this way.

Times have changed. In the past, patients generally had one or two medical problems; now they have five, ten, or even twenty. There were fewer diagnostic tests in the "old days." As technology has advanced, the array of diagnostic decisions has grown exponentially. The number of treatment options has also grown significantly. These options include those for medications that correct physiologic abnormalities and those for procedures that can repair or replace malfunctioning body parts. Preventive care protocols for healthy patients are also more complex—and they change frequently and sometimes conflict with each other. The process of managing more complex patients in more complex settings is further complicated by changes in information management. The EHR has replaced the paper chart, bringing both advantages and disadvantages.

Because of the increasing cost of running a solo practice, most physicians now practice in groups. As small, single-specialty groups have found it challenging to negotiate contracts and manage new payment mechanisms effectively, they have sold their practices to larger groups that are often affiliated with a hospital. Hospitals have seen a massive expansion of diagnostic options, medication choices, and interventional capabilities with scopes and catheters that can do amazing things, all requiring new skills, new or expanded facilities, and new, more complicated billing codes.

All this change has happened with relatively little proactive planning for the impact on the physicians and nurses who do the work. Each change has been incremental, simply added to the workflow present at the time it was introduced, resulting in a "new normal" process that was a bit, but not dramatically, different from before.

Most health care workplaces have not been deliberatively designed to be reliable, to take into account human factors, to engage the workforce, or to create an environment of respect for the worker. In the past most physicians coped with the flawed system through sheer perseverance, their own internal resilience, their connection to the reasons they became a doctor, their ability to re-energize with time away from work, and their ability to control the workplace sufficiently to develop work-arounds to overcome the barriers to care that they encountered on a daily basis.

Today, the daily barriers and frustrations wear a doctor down. The following are just a few of many actual examples of these confounding obstacles to efficient patient care:

- A change in the EHR requires 20 more clicks and 30 more seconds of time for something that previously took 5 seconds and a quick signature; and it happens 60 times a day.
- A patient with 5 chronic diseases and 12 medications was discharged from the hospital, and the new medication plan is not available when the patient shows up for her follow-up appointment one week later.
- A transport stretcher doesn't work properly while rushing a dying patient to the cath lab for a life-saving procedure.
- The waiting room in the emergency department is full because a backlog of patients waiting to be admitted to the hospital hinders the staff's ability to treat newly arriving patients.
- The EKG machine is still broken two weeks after the unit manager submitted a work order for its repair.

We could fill the rest of the book with more such examples of the workplace frustrations that physicians face daily.

The frustrations have escalated to the point that they have overwhelmed most physicians' traditional coping mechanisms. Physicians no longer feel satisfaction and joy in their practice, and many develop symptoms of burnout. More and more physicians are finding they cannot sustain their previous level of practice over the long term.

For this reason, addressing workplace interventions is essential for preventing burnout. Wellness programs and other interventions focused on increasing physician resilience and decreasing the stresses that individual physicians bring to their practice are simply insufficient. And to design effective workplace interventions, it is important to understand the specific factors within the practice setting that sap the joy from practice and lead to burnout.

## RESEARCH ON BURNOUT DRIVERS IN THE WORKPLACE

Burnout has been defined as "a syndrome that develops in response to problematic relationships between employees and their workplaces." (Leiter 2014) The research literature suggests that misalignment, misfit, or imbalance is responsible for these problematic relationships. (Maslach 2008) Maslach and Leiter have identified six domains in which such mismatch leads to burnout among workers in the general population: (Maslach 2001)

- Work overload
- Lack of control
- Insufficient reward
- Breakdown of community
- Absence of fairness
- Conflicting values

## WORK OVERLOAD

When Paul gives presentations to physicians about implementing a Lean management system as a way to prevent burnout, he starts with a short film clip to capture the essence of what it feels like to practice medicine today. The clip shows a hamster running on a wheel that is accelerating. The unfortunate rodent runs faster and faster, but can't keep up. Eventually, he spins around with the wheel and falls off. The reaction in the room is usually a mixture of laughter and resignation. Physicians identify with the outpaced hamster all too well. They understand at a visceral level that the current system takes highly trained, mission-driven professionals and places them in work environments that make it almost impossible for almost anyone to succeed.

Research by Maslach and Leiter identified work demands that "exceed human limits" as a predictor of worker burnout. (Maslach 2008) The researchers place the onus of this mismatch on the workplace, not the worker. "In their scramble for increased productivity, organizations push people beyond what they can sustain. [The increased workload impacts workers] in three ways—it is more intense, it demands more time, and it is more complex. Not surprisingly, relief is hard to find." (Maslach 2000)

We see all three aspects of increased workload in health care today. They are interrelated and have a mutual impact on each other.

**Greater intensity**. The decrease in reimbursement per relative value unit (RVU)[1] incentivizes organizations to produce more RVUs per day in order to maintain current revenues. The expenses of running the business, such as staffing, supplies, medications, and rent, continue to rise. The combination of decreasing revenue and increasing expense per RVU result in the pressure to see more patients with fewer resources, making the work more intense.

**More time-demanding**. For many reasons, the current work of patient care demands more time per patient. Patients have more chronic conditions today than in the past, and each condition needs attention. In most cases, entering new data into the EHR takes longer than dictating or scribbling a handwritten note. External mandates and quality initiatives mean there are more required tasks for each patient, such as ensuring that the medical, social, and family history is updated in the record; that medication lists are reconciled; and that follow-up testing, referrals, and treatments are authorized and scheduled. Time demands are exacerbated if organizational leaders decide, when faced with reducing reimbursements, to maintain operating margins by downsizing support staff, which puts a greater burden on physicians to complete non-clinical or menial tasks.

**Greater complexity**. Patient care today is more complex, as patients present with an increasing number of diagnoses. More diagnoses mean more diagnostic tests, which in turn require more decisions about which tests to perform and in which order; more medications, which increases the risk of adverse drug interactions; and more specialty consultations. In part because of the increasing complexity of patient care and treatment options, most payers require prior authorization for expensive medications and some high-cost diagnostic or interventional procedures. Obtaining the authorization often requires physicians to speak with a nurse or clerk at the insurance company. The interchange can take as long as 30 minutes on the phone per authorization—time diverted from patient care or other clerical tasks.

---

1 The RVU system is an attempt to equitably account for the variation in the intensity and demand of work done across all specialties, from primary care to neurosurgery.

The degree of efficiency in the workplace may also affect an organization's ability to attract and retain clinical staff. As Patricia A. Gabow, MD, former CEO of Denver Health, phrased it, "People don't want to work in a train wreck."

## LACK OF CONTROL

The research of Maslach and Leiter has demonstrated that a lack of personal control of the work environment is an important predictor of burnout. (Maslach 2008) For physicians, being in control of the work environment includes the degree to which they are able to make individual decisions about practice setting, days and hours worked, length of appointments, rooming procedures, and other aspects of patient care. Lack of control over the way a physician spends his or her time can directly affect the risk of burnout. Research has shown that physicians have a lower rate of burnout if they spend 10 to 20 percent of their work week in the area of focus (for example, teaching, research, or direct patient care) that is most personally meaningful to them. (Shanafelt 2009)

Physicians have held professional autonomy as one of their most important values, and for good reason. They undergo rigorous training, engage in ongoing education, and complete certification requirements to ensure they are prepared to make life-and-death decisions in high-stakes settings. Although many aspects of care delivery can be standardized, situations will always exist in which a physician's clinical judgment is paramount.

In years past, physician autonomy over the practice environment and decisions affecting patient care and their practice environment was a given. Recent changes in health care have diminished physicians' sense of professional autonomy. Increasingly, physicians are expected to be engaged participants of interdisciplinary care teams. Instead of acting autonomously, they are expected to collaborate—with patients, with support staff, and with hospital administrators. This move toward collaborative caregiving is a positive change that is long overdue. However, as with any change, losses accompany the gains.

Given that the profession requires a degree of latitude to make urgent decisions in varied circumstances and having earned the right to professional autonomy through training, ongoing education, and certification, many physicians feel dismayed, devalued, or angered by the loss of autonomy. After all, it was, in part, autonomy and individual achievement that attracted many physicians to the profession in the first place.

The trend of moving from having a solo practice to being an employee of a health care organization has also affected physicians' control over practice decisions. Many physicians feel they have made a Faustian bargain when they shift from being the owner of a small business to becoming an employee in a large corporation; they join a larger group to free themselves from the burden of the growing financial risks associated with running a small practice but must abdicate some degree of autonomy and control. A quick perusal of online forums illustrates this conflict. A common theme in blog posts about physician burnout is the sense that administrators are in charge and that physicians must accept the decisions made by others about their practice, the pace and hours of the daily schedule, the number and type of support staff, the equipment and supplies, and the number of exam rooms available to them. Physicians are vocal in these forums about the degree of their discontent.

According to Mark Graban, Lean consultant and vice president of improvement and innovation services for the software company KaiNexus, many of the physicians in the organizations he is asked to help feel the loss of autonomy very acutely. "Autonomy at work is an important expectation for health care professionals that is not present to the same degree in the manufacturing settings where Lean was developed. What is the same is the sense that workers in traditionally managed manufacturing and health care settings feel they cannot make a difference in the workplace."

In some instances, physicians' responses to the loss of autonomy are detrimental to effective care delivery. For example, a doctor may:

- Choose hours of practice for his or her own convenience that conflict with the function of the office or hospital flow
- Adopt individualized processes to schedule, prepare, or treat patients that create unnecessary variation among a group of colleagues

- Demand that he or she have special equipment or supplies that offer no additional benefit but add to the complexity and financial burden of the organization in which he or she works

The frustration that many physicians feel at the loss of autonomy and control over their work sometimes presents as an intense focus on the insufficiency of the rewards of their work.

## INSUFFICIENT REWARD

According to research by Maslach and Leiter, lack of rewards is a key driver of professional burnout. (Maslach 2008) For physicians, the adequacy of financial and non-financial rewards directly affects their daily experience in the workplace. Insufficient rewards can heighten physicians' stress related to personal finances, exacerbate other daily frustrations, and promote a sense of being disrespected. Insufficient rewards can drive physicians' decisions about how much they participate in improvement projects, how actively they choose to pursue leadership positions, and whether or not they stay at an organization. We'll discuss financial rewards in this section. Physicians are also driven by non-financial rewards, which we'll discuss in the next chapter.

**Financial rewards**. Physicians, like other professionals, make their career choice based in part on the anticipated rewards—financial and otherwise. Professionals, and physicians in particular, spend years in training, diverting time and financial resources from other potential investments and sacrificing financial gain in the first decade of their adult lives.

---

## COMPENSATION MODELS

Health care organizations vary in their approaches to compensation. Some hospitals and physician groups pay their physicians a salary—a flat amount based on specialty and percentage of a full-time equivalent (FTE) that the physician works. Others pay based on productivity, measuring the volume of work that the physician provides, often in relative value units (RVUs). Some compensation models include a mixture of base salary and productivity. Alternative forms of compensation are becoming more common. These include payment for taking call, performance bonuses, and payment for administrative work.

**Pay for call.** Pay for taking call has been offered by some hospitals for a while; for others it is a relatively new phenomenon. Such pay has become an increasingly contentious issue in many hospitals, as some specialists are charging higher and higher fees for providing this vital service. In the past, being on call for other physicians was considered an integral aspect of the physician's role; additional pay for taking call was not generally expected. However, in response to reduced reimbursement, physicians began looking for additional sources of income, including pay for call.

**Performance bonuses.** Performance bonuses are an attempt to reward physicians for achieving specific objectives. These can work if properly structured, that is, if they are focused on meaningful aspects of patient care, designed to be achievable, and scaled to be worth the effort. Too often bonuses are not well-structured and cause more discord and disruption than benefit. In fact, performance rewards can backfire. As Daniel H. Pink eloquently explained in *Drive: The Surprising Truth About What Motivates Us*, for work that involves mechanical skills or straightforward tasks, increasing financial rewards has a positive effect on motivation. (Pink 2011) However, for work that involves cognitive skills or a degree of creative thinking, like that of physicians, as long as a professional is paid enough that money is not a significant obstacle; additional rewards will decrease the intrinsic motivation to perform well.

**Pay for administrative work.** Pay for providing administrative services to a hospital is the third form of alternative compensation.

Most health systems pay physicians an hourly rate for various functions, including serving on committees that are vital to patient care services, attending medical staff meetings, participating in training to learn how to use the new EHR system, and participating in improvement activities. The rate is determined by the "fair market value" based on prevailing norms. If the rate is the same for primary care physicians and specialists, the latter may find the rate unfair, because they earn a higher hourly rate than primary care physicians when providing patient care.

———

Most physicians enter the wage-earning phase of their lives in their late twenties or early thirties—even later if they are pursuing subspecialty training. By this age, many non-physicians have established their professional lives, purchased a home, and started accruing retirement savings. In contrast, when physicians enter the working world, many are saddled with $300,000 or more of education debt, have little or no equity in a home, and have not begun saving for retirement.

Financially, then, physicians have a lot of catching up to do. They may expect, or even need, to see high financial returns to extricate themselves from education debt and attain the lifestyle of most working professionals. Outsiders may assume that physicians' salaries are higher than those of most other professions and that they are well compensated for their work. In the past, this was largely true. Now, however, several factors have diminished physicians' take-home pay, including, most prominently, insurers lowering the reimbursement per RVU. Physicians have responded by increasing the number of patients seen per day; finding other sources of income, such as ownership of ambulatory surgery centers; pursuing higher pay for call coverage; or finding ways to cope with the reduced income.

For many physicians, a widening gap exists between the financial rewards of the job and the effort required for the work they do. This gap is most evident for primary care physicians (PCPs). PCPs have lower salaries than specialists and in many cases have more intense work demands. (Medscape 2016) It has been said that as the pie gets smaller, table manners get worse. With the increasing cost and productivity pressures, it is not uncommon for conflicts to erupt among physicians in medical groups about the compensation differences between different specialists.

**Non-financial rewards.** <u>Patients' gratitude.</u> Another important reward for physicians is patients' expressions of gratitude. Clinicians often receive verbal or tangible gifts from patients and their families. Following successful orthopedic or cardiac surgery, patients feel significantly better and are usually grateful to the surgeon who performed the procedure. It's common to see patients bring their surgeon a homemade gift or a bottle of wine to express their gratitude. PCPs enjoy the fruits of meaningful long-term relationships with patients, although the rewards may not come as quickly as those received by the surgeon for the more rapid improvements that follow surgery. Paul changed work locations several times in his clinical career and was consistently moved by the special effort patients made to thank him for being their family physician and let him know how much he would be missed.

Expressions of gratitude to both surgeons and primary care physicians are becoming less frequent as corporate approaches to medicine become more common, as non-clinical tasks increasingly impinge on meaningful physician-patient relationships, and as the physician workforce becomes more mobile. Physicians—who like other clinicians are drawn to medicine because of a desire to help others—feel acutely the loss of the non-financial rewards of patient care.

<u>Recognition.</u> Another valued non-financial reward for physicians is recognition by the organization for a job well done. Today, with the strained relationships between clinicians and administration that are evident in many organizations, physicians may be recognized less often for their contributions to the enterprise and to patients and their families. The failure to recognize the important achievements of physicians can lead to their feeling devalued or disrespected.

Bob Chapman, CEO of the Barry-Wehmiller, a global equipment and engineering company, writes of the importance of workers feeling valued by employers in *Everybody Matters: The Extraordinary Power of Caring for Your People Like Family.* In our interview with Chapman, he emphasized the degree to which workers don't feel valued at their workplace. As he told us, "The majority—88 percent—of people feel they work for an organization that does not care about them. Yet we know that workers that feel 'they care about me' provide better service. This applies in business but it also applies in the military and to health care."

Chapman's statement about the scope of the problem is corroborated by a 2015 industry-conducted survey of more than 2,000 physicians. The survey showed that 82 percent felt that their administration offered no help in dealing with stress and burnout. (VITAL 2015) The sense of not being valued is antithetical to building collaboration, engagement, and alignment with organizational goals. Combined with other burnout drivers, it can sap a physician's resilience to burnout and his or her joy in practice.

## BREAKDOWN OF COMMUNITY

The research on professional burnout conducted by Maslach and Leiter identified breakdown of community as another key driver of burnout. (Maslach 2001) The social context in which burnout develops is important. As Maslach concluded, "Unfortunately, some jobs isolate people from each other, or make social contact impersonal. However, what is most destructive of community is chronic and unresolved conflict with others on the job." (Maslach 2001)

**Diminished contact with colleagues.** Most physicians thrive on interpersonal interaction. They may not tend toward extroversion, but most deeply value connecting with their patients and collaborating with their colleagues and support staff. This human connection is an important element in most physicians' attraction to the work in the first place. Often the physicians, other clinicians, and support staff in a practice or a clinical department will develop a deep sense of camaraderie and esprit de corps as they are united by the common goal of providing great care to the patients they serve. Collaboration around a common goal is a core feature of the culture of many health care organizations.

However, recent changes in care delivery have weakened this camaraderie. Foremost among these changes are the pressure to be more productive with fewer resources; the increase in specialization, with fewer physicians practicing in both the hospital and office setting; and a profound, EHR-driven shift in how clinicians review information and communicate with each other. For many clinicians, these shifts have resulted in increased isolation, less positive connections with co-workers, and increased conflict and tension in the workplace.

As a result of the pressure to be more productive, physicians' down time has largely evaporated. In the past, physicians often had time to discuss the latest changes in treatment recommendations with colleagues or review a challenging case with a peer. At one time, the doctors' lounge at the hospital was a vibrant place where colleagues connected several times daily, often exchanging valuable clinical information or sharing news of their recent vacation and the latest achievements of their children. This is no longer the case. Now many physicians strive to keep up with the demands of documenting clinic notes and responding to inbox messages. Fewer physicians work within the hospital today, and those who do are often so busy that they spend little time connecting with colleagues.

These changes have had a profound impact on physicians' sense of community. Robert Wachter of the University of California, San Francisco, eloquently describes these changes in *The Digital Doctor: Hope, Hype, and Harm at the Dawn of Medicine's Computer Age.* He writes, "Walk around the ER and you'll see them: doctors and nurses, just inches away from each other, staring at their computers without exchanging a word." (Wachter 2015) When one looks around the hospital wards for physicians, they are most likely to be in the workstation area, typing in their electronic orders and progress notes.

Radiologists are among the hardest hit by these changes. In the past, morning rounds included an obligatory visit by members of the care team to the radiology suite, where the radiologist would personally review the films with them. Now clinicians no longer take the time to venture into the imaging department; they simply view the digital images on the ward. The radiologists toil away, reading image after image as quickly as possible and trying to keep up with the increased volume of studies ordered by hospitalists and emergency physicians who, not knowing the patients personally as was frequently the case when PCPs saw their own patients in the hospital, now order more imaging studies to firm up their diagnoses and assessments.

In the past, when a physician requested a specialty consultation, he or she would personally call the specialist before placing the order in the chart. The specialist would briefly review the case for its appropriateness and request any relevant information and tests to be done in preparation for the consultation. With the decline of personal relationships between clinicians, it is now common for the consultation to be requested as an order in the EHR without any discussion between the consultant and the ordering physician.

The lost sense of community among physicians has ripple effects throughout the health care system. In his work, Paul has seen firsthand how the weakening of personal connections and reduction in direct communication can have negative secondary effects, such as longer lengths of stay, higher costs, unnecessary procedures, potential medication errors, and lower quality of care. The lost sense of community is exacerbated by conflicts between the physicians' personal and professional responsibilities.

**Perceived lack of respect.** Feeling respected is critically important to one's sense of identity and dignity. In contrast, feeling disrespected can ignite intense emotions and spark angry or even violent behavior. As Kerry Patterson and his co-authors wrote in *Crucial Conversations: Tools for Talking When Stakes Are High,* "Respect is like air, if you take it away, it's all people can think about." (Patterson 2012) Physicians are highly trained professionals who tend to value autonomy and the ability to make decisions independently. They generally expect to be treated with respect. Behavior on the part of leaders that physicians interpret as disrespect can cause intense negative reactions to flare up.

Perceived lack of respect can also affect relationships between physicians and other clinicians or staff. Monica Broome, MD, assistant professor at University of Miami Miller School of Medicine, has observed this connection in her work as a master trainer for the Institute for Healthcare Communication. "Respect is so important, yet people tend to underestimate its significance. Then they miss opportunities for making a positive connection by simply showing respect." She believes that lack of respect among clinicians combined with underutilization of their professional skills can lead to difficulty connecting with colleagues, less effective clinical teams, and a failure to achieve the gratification that comes from using one's skills to the best of one's abilities. These problems then lead to burnout among physicians.

In speaking with physicians, we've learned that many today feel disrespected by a variety of parties in the health care system: patients, their family members, nurses, other clinical staff, agents at health insurance companies, and others. However, the source of disrespect that seems to frustrate physicians the most is leaders of health care provider organizations, especially CEOs. Physicians have described blatant cases of disrespect by CEOs. Disrespect most commonly surfaces during disputes that have high personal stakes for physicians, such as the negotiation of the terms of a joint venture between the hospitals and physicians, of call coverage frequency and compensation, or of the acquisition of the physicians' practice by the hospital. Although such conflicts are not common, they can lead to a negative culture of distrust between the two most influential leadership groups in a health care system.

Also important are the less-blatant cases—for example, the unintended disrespect a physician experiences because of the actions and decisions of the CEO. For instance, a CEO, under pressure to improve the health system's performance metrics, might push physicians to improve without communicating why the performance gap exists or working collaboratively with the physicians to decide how best to close the gap. Physicians feel a profound sense of disrespect from the failure to involve them in key decisions that affect their daily practice and about which they have sophisticated, firsthand knowledge. A CEO may have more business training and acumen than most physicians, but he or she is less likely to understand the details of operations (that is, workflows) that are responsible for the underperformance he or she is trying to address.

Physicians who feel disrespected by CEOs will often respond in one of three ways. First, they may discredit the data. Physicians are trained as scientists to doubt hypotheses until substantial proof exists; discrediting data is second nature. Given the many problems with the way most performance metrics are generated, such doubt is a predictable response. Second, they may challenge whether the concept behind the metric is valid. For example, when being assessed on patient satisfaction scores, physicians might focus on the possibility that low scores may reflect better patient care, such as when a physician rejects patient requests for unnecessary tests or treatment. Third, physicians may become adamant in their demands for the resources needed to achieve the desired outcome, such as additional staff, expanded facilities, new equipment, a slower pace, or higher compensation. Although physicians' requests often reflect a true need for additional resources, the passion behind the request may reflect underlying anger related to feeling disrespected.

Steven Beeson, MD, an author and the founder of The Physician Effectiveness Project at PracticingExcellence.com, explains this dynamic as "placing a metric above the mission." He told us, "As physicians, we are here to change the lives of our patients. Metrics are the quantitative proof of the mission, but they can't become the mission." When metrics trump the mission, it demoralizes physicians.

In contrast, we have seen that when a leader treats physicians with respect, presenting problems in a way that engages physicians and enables collaboration between administration and the medical staff, the dynamic is dramatically different. Collaborating to solve a shared problem is a profound way to show respect.

**Interprofessional conflict and disconnect**. Interprofessional conflict and disconnect is an example of the breakdown of community, which is a known driver of burnout. Such conflict can occur when discord erupts among physicians in a medical group or between administrators and medical staff. "Turf wars" are a major source of conflict and can emerge due to disagreements about which specialty should be treating which conditions or has the right to perform certain procedures as well as about which specialty should be responsible for which aspects of patient care.

Disagreements over privileges to perform procedures are common. Such disagreements carry high stakes because they impact compensation as well as a physician's sense of self-worth. Primary care physicians have experienced a steady decrease in the range of procedures they perform and the patients they care for. Many years ago, they would deliver babies, perform surgeries, provide intensive care, and cover the emergency room. As the number of specialists and complexity of care has increased, PCPs have relinquished these activities. In some cases, this was the PCP's choice, but in others it was the result of actions by specialists to deny the PCPs those privileges.

This is not just a PCP versus specialist issue. Specialists also have seen changes in privileging. For example, vascular surgeons and interventional radiologists were initially the primary specialists using catheters to open narrowed carotid and femoral arteries. Cardiologists generally used the technique only in the heart. Increasingly, though, cardiologists are moving onto the turf of vascular surgeons and interventional radiologists by performing procedures in the neck and legs as well.

## ABSENCE OF FAIRNESS

The research of Maslach and Leiter identified absence of fairness as a key predictor of burnout. (Maslach 2008) Physicians see themselves as working as hard as they can in a workplace full of barriers that make their already challenging job even more difficult. It's easy to see why a physician in this situation would be quick to notice a lack of fairness in the workplace. The salaries of health system executives are an increasing source of frustration for physicians. Many physicians feel that they are working harder and contributing more than the hospital CEO, whose salary is widely known because it is published in the media every year.

Physicians find this mismatch particularly galling, as the same CEO may have made it more difficult for the physician to meet the system-dictated performance expectations by deciding to cut the support staff that the doctor relies on, change the brand of an implant the physician prefers, or take other unpopular, cost-cutting actions ostensibly needed to keep the hospital financially stable.

Fairness issues can also erupt between physicians. Medical staff leaders have a responsibility to ensure that physicians in their hospital are competent to care for their patients. In some circumstances these leaders are competing for patients with the physicians whose hospital privileges they approve or deny. Despite attempts to make the process objective, there are always gray areas of subjectivity that can cause a physician to feel that he or she was unfairly denied hospital privileges. Although such cases are rare, Paul has personally witnessed physician leaders using their positions to attempt to limit privileges inappropriately to achieve a political or financial objective. For example, in one instance, a physician who had an ongoing dispute with a CEO challenged the CEO's competence in a medical staff meeting. The CEO retaliated by limiting the physician's privileges at the hospital, citing disruptive behavior and poor quality of care as the reason. In several cases, actions on the part of an executive that were perceived to be unfair by a physician led to legal challenges that placed significant psychological stress on all involved.

## CONFLICTING VALUES

Perhaps the most strongly held value common to all physicians is the desire to provide the highest quality care to every patient. Many of the physicians we interviewed discussed the challenge of staying true to this value in a world in which the realities of limited resources drive physicians to make moral judgments every day regarding care. A misalignment between the values of physicians and those of organizational leaders is reflected in a number of the conflicts we have already mentioned, such as administrators demanding higher levels of performance while reducing the level of support staff and physicians not having adequate time in appointments to connect with their patients or address all of the patients' needs.

In this highly volatile, competitive landscape, health system leaders make strategic decisions that, by their nature, will not please everyone. In some cases, physicians may disagree with the strategic plans of their employer. Such conflicts are exacerbated when the leaders profess to follow one strategy, but take actions inconsistent with it. For example, a leader may express a desire to move from volume- to value-based payment mechanisms and yet, in order to maintain an influx of fee-for-service revenue, purchase additional MRIs or add operating rooms. To physicians who are not privy to all aspects of the decision-making process, this incongruence is a source of discord.

∭

In this chapter, we've described the workplace factors predictive of burnout among professionals in the general population. In the next chapter, we'll discuss some additional factors that emerged as predictors of burnout in studies of physicians.

# REFERENCES

Aryee S, Sun LY, Chen ZXG, Debrah YA. Abusive supervision and contextual performance: the mediating role of emotional exhaustion and the moderating role of work unit structure. *Manag Org Rev.* 2008;4:393–411.

Bakker AB, Demerouti E. The job demands-resources model: state of the art. *J Manag Psychol.* 2007;22:309–328.

Breevaart K, Bakker AB, Hetland J, Hetland H. The influence of constructive and destructive leadership behaviors on follower burnout. In: Leiter MP, Bakker AB, Maslach C, eds. *Burnout at Work: A Psychological Perspective.* New York: Psychological Press. 2014:102–121.

Gregory ST, Menser T. Burnout among primary care physicians: a test of the areas of work life model. *J Healthcare Manag.* 2015;60(2):133–148.

Leiter M, Maslach C. Interventions to prevent and alleviate burnout. In: Leiter MP, Bakker AB, Maslach C, eds. *Burnout at Work: A Psychological Perspective.* New York: Psychological Press. 2014:145–167.

Linzer M, Manwell LB, Williams ES, et al. Working conditions in primary care: physician reactions and care quality. *Ann Intern Med.* 2009;151(1):28–36.

Maslach C, Leiter MP. Early predictors of job burnout and engagement. *J Appl Psychol.* 2008;93(3):498–512.

Maslach C, Schaufeli WB, Leiter M. Job burnout. *Annu. Rev. Psychol.* 2001;52:397–422.

Maslach C, Leiter M. *The Truth About Burnout: How Organizations Cause Personal Stress and What to Do About It.* San Francisco: Jossey-Bass. 2000.

Medscape physicians compensation report. 2016. Available at: http://www.medscape.com/features/slideshow/compensation/2016/public/overview#page=2. Accessed July 8, 2016.

Patterson K, Grenny J, McMillan R, Switzler A. *Crucial Conversations: Tools for Talking When Stakes Are High.* New York: McGraw-Hill. 2012.

Pink DH. *Drive: The Surprising Truth About What Motivates Us.* New York: Riverhead Books. 2011.

Shanafelt TD, Gorringe G, Menaker R, et al. Impact of organizational leadership on physician burnout and satisfaction. *Mayo Clin Proc.* 2015;90(4):432–440.

Shanafelt TD, West CP, Sloan JA, et al. Career fit and burnout among academic faculty. *Arch Intern Med.* 2009;169(10):990–995.

Tepper BJ. Is there a relationship between burnout and objective performance? A critical review of 16 studies. *Work Stress.* 2000;43:178–190.

VITAL WorkLife & Cejka Search. 2015 physician stress and burnout report. Available at: http://vitalworklife.com/wp-content/uploads/2015/02/2015-Stress-Burnout-Survey-Report-02-15-with-links.pdf. Accessed June 28, 2016.

Wachter R. *The Digital Doctor: Hope, Hype, and Harm at the Dawn of Medicine's Computer Age.* New York: McGraw-Hill. 2015:77.

# CHAPTER 5
## Workplace Drivers of Burnout for Physicians

*At one site with one hundred fifty or so physicians, we were hemorrhaging five or six doctors per year. Now that we've improved the care teams, we're attracting six physicians a year.*
—Paul Grundy, MD, MPH, global director of health care transformation for IBM, personal communication, April 25, 2016

*People don't want to work in a train wreck. They want to work where it's transparent and fair, and where they're acknowledged.*
—Patricia A. Gabow, MD, former CEO of Denver Health, personal communication, December 1, 2015

As we described in Chapter 4, six factors drive burnout among professionals. These provide a starting point for considering the causes of the burnout crisis among physicians. However, researchers studying burnout in physicians have discovered several additional factors specific to the physician's workplace that increase the risk of burnout.

Mark Linzer and his research team at the University of Minnesota have studied physician burnout for several decades. One of their early studies, funded by the Agency for Healthcare Research and Quality, identified factors in the workplace conditions of physicians that increase the risk of adverse physician reactions (stress, burnout, dissatisfaction, and intent to leave). The predictors of burnout included the following (Linzer 2009):

- Chaos
- Time pressure
- Lack of control
- Misalignment of values with the organization

In other research, Linzer identified an additional factor as predictive of physician burnout: work-home interference. (Linzer 2001)

Tait Shanafelt and his research team at the Mayo Clinic have conducted research on physician burnout that has provided nationwide data on prevalence, demographics, and risk factors. In a 2016 presentation that was part of a joint Mayo Clinic–*New England Journal of Medicine* Catalyst project, Shanafelt identified six causes of physician burnout. (Shanafelt 2016) These are the following:

- Work overload
- Inefficiencies and undue clerical burden
- Loss of control
- Work-life imbalance
- Loss of meaning in work
- Conflicting values

Substantial overlap exists between the drivers of burnout identified by Maslach for the general population and those identified by Linzer and Shanafelt for physicians. In the last chapter, we discussed the factors shared by physicians and the general population, namely, work overload, lack of control, work-life imbalance, loss of meaning in work, and conflicting values. In this chapter we'll cover the factors identified by Linzer and by Shanafelt that were not identified by research on professional burnout in the general population. These factors include:

- Chaos and inefficiencies
- Undue clerical burden
- Time pressure

- Work-life imbalance
- Loss of meaning in work

We'll cover undue clerical burden briefly in this chapter. Chapter 7 is devoted entirely to the effects of the EHR on physicians.

_____

## RESEARCH ON DRIVERS OF PHYSICIAN DISSATISFACTION AND BURNOUT

Kristine Olsen, MD, MS, a health services researcher and assistant professor of clinical medicine at Yale School of Medicine, is currently studying the correlates of physician satisfaction and burnout among 4,300 physicians affiliated with Yale–New Haven Health System. Her research has identified physician satisfaction as a proxy for how well a physician is able to function within a health system to provide patient-centered care. The factors that predict satisfaction fall into two categories: practice management and clinical decision making. The factors for practice management include:

- Quality of relationships with leaders, staff, and other care providers
- Mission alignment with leaders
- Teamwork with staff
- Communication and coordination with other care providers
- Reputation and competitiveness of the practice, presence of fair markets
- Absence of "hassle factors" (that is, the tasks required by third parties to procure goods and services for patients, including ease of use of the communications system and activities related to seeking preapprovals, compliance, billing, coding, collections, documentation, and data collection)
- Absence of "hustle factors" (that is, the increased pressure to be more productive, seeing more patients in less time while

addressing more tasks and caring for patients with more comorbidities and complexity with little support)

Just one factor relates to clinical decision making:

- Minimal interference with patient-centered clinical decision making and the patient-physician relationship (that is, ease in obtaining the services that are best for their patients)

Her current research is focused on supporting physicians' work through more efficient workplaces, which requires addressing the effects of clerical interference (for example, the EHR burden); through engaging physicians' perspectives in innovation and management; and through fostering alignment between leaders and physicians.

_____

## CHAOS AND INEFFICIENCIES

Linzer's research identified workplace chaos as one of the key predictors of physician stress, burnout, and intention to leave. (Linzer 2009) A recent analysis of the data showed that physicians in clinics with chaotic work environments had significantly more stress and burnout and a higher likelihood of leaving the practice within two years. (Perez 2015) These clinics also had significantly more missed opportunities to provide preventative services and had significantly higher rates of medical errors.

Our experience and that of many of the physicians we interviewed confirmed the importance of workplace chaos in the development of burnout. Diane identified workplace chaos as the most important factor in the burnout that led her to leave clinical practice. Craig Albanese, MD, MBA, senior vice president and chief operating officer at New York-Presbyterian/Morgan Stanley Children's Hospital and Sloane Hospital for Women, pointed to the chaos and unstable work environment as the driver of his increasing interest in taking on administrative roles. He sensed that "there's got to be a better way." According to John Toussaint,

MD, CEO of the ThedaCare Center for Healthcare Value, the workplace prior to implementing a Lean transformation at ThedaCare was replete with inefficiencies. "Physicians, nurses, and administrators and everybody else were all running around like chickens with their heads cut off because all the processes were chaos. There was no standard work. You did it one way on Monday, another way on Tuesday, and a third way on Wednesday. There was no predictability."

Toussaint told us that he and other leaders hypothesized that if they created predictability through standard work, the organization could focus on defect identification and problem-solving at the source. This approach, they believed, would lead to a more stable environment for caregivers and for patients. He described an informal study he did early in the organization's Lean journey. He shadowed a nurse for a week with a stopwatch. The results? Three and a half hours of an eight-hour shift were spent searching for supplies. "It was the same for physicians in the office. What they needed was not in the room when they needed it. They didn't have the information they needed to make decisions. Process after process was so fundamentally broken; it's understandable why people were very stressed out."

In an interview, James P. Womack, PhD, founder and senior advisor to the Lean Enterprise Institute, described a conversation he had with several residents after delivering a presentation at a prestigious academic hospital. He asked the trainees, "What have you learned about medicine?" One said, "Nothing works, so I've learned how to do workarounds." The fundamental flaw with work-arounds is that they don't fix the underlying error-prone and inefficient processes. These work-arounds can make practice feel a bit like a revolving door. As Gene Lindsey, formerly at Atrius Health, put it, "It became obvious to me that some things were beyond our ability to change as individual providers. We saw the same problems every day, and just because you solved them one day didn't mean they wouldn't come back, because the solutions were work-arounds. They didn't solve the real problems."

Lindsey told us that at one institution in which he practiced for many years, two awards were given annually to recognize clinicians for stellar patient care. "It occurred to me that they should have been called 'Band-Aid awards,' because the system was so dysfunctional it required heroic efforts to provide care." He noted that such efforts cost the physicians in "personal time and a cascade of other losses." The physicians were willing to make the effort, but the dysfunctional system was the root cause of these sacrifices. He said, "It's perverse not to recognize that a lot of their effort was wasted human effort."

Why are practice environments so chaotic and inefficient? In a setting in which errors can have devastating consequences that can be fatal, why are so many workflows inconsistent and unreliable? The simple answer is that the current practice environments were not consciously designed to be efficient and reliable. They developed over time, as multiple improvement initiatives (or external mandates or the personal preference of individual clinicians) changed workflows. The cumulative changes occurred without a careful assessment of the collective impact. The result is the chaos in which most physicians practice every day in both the hospital and office settings. As Robert Wachter of University of California, San Francisco, described it to us, "We have created jobs that are undoable. We have not given a moment's thought to rethinking the world in which physicians provide care."

A common source of chaos in the clinical workplace is the inefficiency of both administrative and care processes. Physicians perform highly technical work that involves significant quality and safety risks. When physicians express fear that they will inadvertently harm a patient, this anxiety is often reflective of a chaotic workplace. Physicians know what to do, but the disorganized, dysfunctional, unpredictable practice environment in which they work makes it difficult, if not impossible, to do the right thing consistently. Attempting to predict and avoid medical errors in such an environment requires a high degree of vigilance, which is unsustainable in the long term.

According to Hereford, this level of vigilance increases the risk of burnout. "The primary contributing factor to burnout is lack of thoughtful processes and support that avoids hero-level work." We asked Hereford to explain what these processes and support would look like. He told us, "Every ambulatory clinic should have a well-codified prepare-for-visit process. But walk into almost any ambulatory clinic and look for that process, and it is non-existent. Instead, the physician shows up at the appointed time and tries to do his or her best with the summary information in the medical record while trying to engage with the patient. Little wonder it's a stressful encounter. At the end of the visit, there's no well-codified process for the patient exit, follow-up, documentation, or coding. We just expect physicians to function well anyway. It's ridiculous when you say it out loud." Wayne Sotile has seen a direct connection between inefficiency and burnout. He told us that the primary complaint of the physicians and nurses he's worked with is inefficiencies in the work setting.

Lindsey described it this way: "If you step back and look at [burnout symptoms] and get beyond feeling like it is happening because you're a deficient human being, you realize that these things are happening because you're functioning in a system that is inhumane and not designed for anyone's psychological or emotional survival."

Jack Billi, MD, a senior Lean deployment leader who has been a practicing internist at the University of Michigan for 38 years, relayed a story that exemplified workplace inefficiencies and frustrations. A team was using Lean to improve work processes in an obstetrics clinic. During a debrief, Billi asked the team members to describe a change they tested. A team member sheepishly described a small change that had a big impact. Prior to the change, the drawers in the exam tables in each room were occasionally locked, requiring the physician to go find a staff member with a key, often mid-exam. In the debrief with Billi, a department chair described the situation this way: "The difference between a good day and a bad day in clinic are small things like whether that drawer was locked." After a few tests of change, the team had all the locks removed.

According to Billi, it is just this sort of small frustration that saps a clinician's energy reserves. As he put it, "The printer doesn't work. The badge tap-and-go tool on the computer is down, so you have to log in every time you touch the keyboard. There are no translators available when you need one. It's all sand in the gears."

## UNDUE CLERICAL BURDEN

A significant element in the current workload of physicians is clerical tasks that have little to do with the practice of medicine per se. Required data entry and other clerical tasks divert time from patient care and sap physicians' ability to connect with the meaning inherent in their daily work.

In an interview, Christine Sinsky, MD, vice president of professional satisfaction at the American Medical Association and a general internist in Dubuque, Iowa, summed up her observations about the undue clerical burden on physicians, saying, "Burnout results from spending our days doing the wrong things." In her work with the American Medical Association on its core strategic initiative to improve physician career satisfaction and practice sustainability, she receives input from physicians across the country. She told us,

> Physicians despair over the gap between their professional aspirations and what they are able to do in the current socio-technical-regulatory environment. For example, physicians find that technology can, at times, make it harder to interact with their patients in a personal way. The often robotic history recorded in the EHR doesn't always tell patient's story. The value placed on human interactions has been decreased in many care environments. Too often, the tools and regulations result in care that has become transactional, not relational.

In an interview, Rick Dart, MD, PhD, director of the Rocky Mountain Poison and Drug Center and former chief business development officer at Denver Health, described the effects of administrative burdens. He said, "A huge part of physician burnout is physicians come to the role with dreams and expectations, and all of a sudden the world says, 'Wrong. You're not going to spend a lot of time teaching. You're not going to spend a lot of time talking to your patient. You're going to spend a lot of time doing paperwork.' I'm not surprised there's a lot of burnout."

Sue Cejka, a managing partner at Grant Cooper Healthcare and experienced physician recruiter who talks with leaders and physicians nationwide, shared her view with us. She said, "Talk about practicing at the top of your license? This isn't even practicing. It's filling out paperwork. The first thing we need to do [to address burnout] is change this."

She has seen physicians who are proactively addressing the situation, for example, by "experimenting on themselves and their practices" or by studying the cost of a scribe compared to the cost of time lost by the physician typing.

Physician burnout coach Michelle Mudge-Riley sees the toll these burdens take on her clients. "The reason they went into medicine, to offer service and be there for patients, is being compromised by other things getting in the way. The EHR and ICD-10 are contributing factors." Physicians themselves identify administrative tasks, especially data entry, as being a primary cause of burnout. A 2016 Medscape survey found that "too many bureaucratic tasks" was the most commonly identified cause of burnout. (Medscape 2016) The next five most common responses were the following: spending too many hours at work, increasing computerization of practice, insufficient income, feeling like a "cog in a wheel," and maintenance of certification requirements. Many of our interviewees voiced similar perspectives. As Dike Drummond, MD, a physician coach, consultant on physician burnout, and author of *Stop Physician Burnout: What to Do When Working Harder Isn't Working*, told us, "When I ask physicians to list their top five stressors, at least three of them are related to documentation" (personal conversation, January 26, 2016).

The EHR is arguably the most important of the technical and administrative burdens that physicians face today. For this reason, we've devoted Chapter 7 solely to the EHR and its relationship to physician burnout.

## TIME PRESSURE

The increase in workload is related to another key predictor of physician burnout: time pressure. Linzer's research demonstrated that increased time pressure is associated with lower physician job satisfaction. (Linzer 2000) Maslach and Leiter describe the connection between time pressure and the development of burnout symptoms. They write, "Restful moments between events are gone. Each demand rolls without a break into the next. There is no time to catch your breath. Organizations seem to be testing the theory that people can work flat-out forever. But, with no time to recover, people soon find that their exhaustion just builds." (Maslach 2000)

Most physicians who read this quote will relate. They start their day already feeling behind, often with schedules overbooked and electronic inboxes filled with calls, test results, and refill requests. They try to keep on schedule, but patients present to the office with problems that are too numerous or complex to be managed in a 15-minute appointment. In the inpatient setting, unanticipated complications, additional procedures, new admissions, and unexpected consultation requests threaten the physician's ability to finish clinical rounds and complete documentation before scheduled meetings or procedures.

Lunch is a time to catch up. The physician is often completing care for the last scheduled patient in the morning 30 to 60 minutes after the session was scheduled to end, and he or she often spends the remainder of the lunch period returning phone calls and completing the chart notes from the morning. Before the catch-up work from the morning is completed, the afternoon schedule starts with the same futile attempt to stay on schedule.

George Palma at Simpler described a day when, as a practicing neurologist, he experienced this type of time pressure. He said, "It was early evening on the Wednesday before Thanksgiving, and I was on call for our neurology group. At 5:00 p.m., after clinic ended, I realized I had 12 consults to do before I could finish my work day. I thought to myself, 'This doesn't work.'"

Evenings provide little respite. It's common for physicians to get home for dinner with their loved ones only to return to their keyboards for several hours at night, completing visit notes, reviewing test results, and responding to phone messages left by their support staff during the afternoon. In addition, if they are on call, they must also field calls and text messages. Weekends provide some down time but in many cases include four to six hours of catch-up work and time to read the latest journal articles.

The time pressure also can threaten physicians' ability to practice according to their values. As Suzanne Koven, MD, wrote in a 2016 essay in *The New England Journal of Medicine*, "The dilemma I face most often as a primary care doctor…is not [lack of resources like medication]. The commodities I struggle to ration are my own time and emotional energy. Almost every day I see a patient like the woman with diarrhea and I find myself at a crossroads: do I ask her what's really bothering her and risk a time-consuming interaction? Or do I accept what she's saying at face value and risk missing a chance to truly help her?" (Koven 2016)

What is the result of this unrealistic workload and intense time pressure? To maintain a full-time clinical schedule, many physicians need to work 80 or more hours a week. There are several downstream effects of this new reality. Some physicians are developing carpal tunnel syndrome due to excessive keyboarding, which can restrict their ability to see patients and reduce their productivity. Some physicians are opting to work part-time, reducing their incomes and in some cases their health and retirement benefits. Physicians working such demanding hours also have less time for involvement in family activities, placing additional stress on other family members.

Lindsey described the situation this way, summarizing a book by Robert Coles, *The Call of Service: A Witness to Idealism*, that he found helpful during his early clinical career: "You can take any well-meaning soul who is mission driven and turn them into a cynical SOB just by continually asking them to do more than they have the physical energy or emotional resilience to do. It's just a function of exhaustion."

## WORK-LIFE IMBALANCE

Linzer and colleagues have identified work-home interference as an important stressor that can contribute to physician burnout. (Linzer 2001) Although the balance between professional and personal responsibilities is a common source of stress for many working adults, the problem has recently escalated for physicians, outpacing the stress experienced by other working adults. Research from the Mayo Clinic demonstrated that from 2011 to 2014 both burnout and work-life dissatisfaction increased for physicians, but not for a control group of working professionals. (Shanafelt 2015) The study also found that the median number of hours that physicians work continues to exceed that of other professionals by 10 (50 versus 40 hours per week), with 42 percent of physicians working 60 or more hours per week.

The surge in technical and administrative tasks, especially those related to the EHR have had a huge impact on the physician's home life, according to the physicians and health care experts we interviewed. Many physicians spend several additional hours each day working from home, trying to finish up the day's progress notes and address all the patient messages, refill requests, and prior authorizations required by third-party payers.

Technological advances allow us to take work outside the workplace, shifting the expectations for many professions about working during "off" hours. The EHR has extended the reach of work pressures to the physician's home, so there truly is no relief.

The increasing time demands of clinical care have negatively affected the work-life balance and family relationships of many physicians. Physician parents may be able to get home to have dinner with their family, but they then commonly disappear into a home office to continue working. Physicians who are mothers may feel the work-home conflict more acutely because of the continuing imbalance in household responsibilities between men and women in many homes. However, work-life conflict is not unique to women. Montgomery Elmer, MD, a family medicine physician at ThedaCare told us, "I was so busy with work that I had little time to recharge at home with my family or to exercise. I missed out on spending more time at home when my children were young and I regret that."

Linzer shared his observations of work-life conflicts at his organization. The health system had traditionally held a strict policy about the beginning and ending times for the general medicine clinic. The strict policy was a source of significant stress for the many physicians at the clinic who were parents of young children. When the clinic ran late or patients scheduled at the end of the day needed time-consuming follow-up planning, it placed significant stress on these physicians, who often needed to drive across town in rush-hour traffic to pick up a child from daycare or after-school program. The stress level of these physicians was "through the roof," according to Linzer. The organization subsequently revised the clinic policies to allow more flexible start and stop times, and the burnout levels in the clinic improved significantly.

## LOSS OF MEANING IN WORK

The practice of medicine offers many valuable non-monetary rewards. Chief among these is the sense of meaning and joy in practice that physicians experience when serving others in times of need. As Ricardo Guerra, Jr., MD, practicing cardiologist and executive board member at Walnut Hill Medical Center in Dallas, put it, "What we do as physicians is life-changing. It's why we do what we do. We're there at the beginning of life and we're there at the end of life. It's a privilege." Guerra told us that when a small group of physicians was planning to found the hospital more than a decade ago, they saw protecting a sense of meaning and joy as indispensable. "The vision for our new hospital could not be 'We're going to create a highly efficient enterprise that delivers high-quality health care and moves bodies in and out as fast as possible...' No one gets out of bed for that." Similarly, Paul Melinkovich of Denver Health told us, "We all want to work in an environment where people have joy in their work, where we feel like everyone is supporting each other, and where we think we are doing good for our patients."

Because a sense of meaning is at the heart of clinical careers in health care, its loss has a tremendous effect on clinicians. As Sotile described it, "Meaning is an antidote to burnout. Physicians need to do work where they see meaning." Guerra voiced a similar sentiment, saying, "Burnout comes from feeling like a cog in a big machine. If you feel like a commodity, it negates the importance of your work. When you're told that anyone could do what you do, it adds to dissatisfaction and a sense of helplessness." Inefficacy, one of the three symptoms of burnout, reflects this sense of lost meaning.

Research confirms the connection between a lack of meaning in work and the risk of burnout. In a survey of 465 academic physicians in internal medicine, researchers at the Mayo Clinic found that those who spent less than 20 percent of their work time engaged in the aspect of work they found most meaningful (for example, patient care, research, or education) had significantly higher rates of burnout (54 percent vs. 30 percent). (Shanafelt 2009)

Much has been written in the past several years about the erosion of a sense of meaning in work and professional satisfaction and joy in practice. One physician described the cause of the erosion of joy in medicine this way: "[The] increasingly burdensome rules and regulations are making it hard to enjoy medical practice these days...Physicians' jobs are becoming increasingly bureaucratic. This bureaucratization can draw physicians' attention away from the purpose of their work—making patients' lives better." (Ubel 2015) Several initiatives have been developed to understand and address the loss of joy in practice. For example, Sinsky and colleagues conducted on-site assessments of 23 high-performing primary care practices with the express goal of identifying factors that fostered joy and satisfaction in practice. They found that these 23 practices were using a number of innovations to sustain joy in practice, including a shift from a physician-centric model to a team-based strategy. (Sinsky 2013)

$$\iiint$$

Physicians are smart. They see the numerous gaps, barriers, and inefficiencies in their organizations that hamper better care. They find work-arounds when they can, or they work harder. They do their best to function in workplaces that are too often fundamentally broken. Trying so hard in an environment plagued with inefficient processes, confounding policies, and frequent communication gaps is a recipe for burnout.

In the next chapters, we'll look at how the role of leadership, the challenges of the EHR, and the factors external to the health care organization have transformed the practice environment of many physicians into a source of torment and distress.

## REFERENCES

Koven S. The doctor's new dilemma. *N Engl J Med.* 2016;374:608–609.

Linzer M, Konrad TR, Douglas J, et al. Managed care, time pressure, and physician job satisfaction: results from the physician worklife study. *J Gen Intern Med.* 2000;15(7):441–450.

Linzer M, Manwell LB, Williams ES, et al. Working conditions in primary care: physician reactions and care quality. *Ann Intern Med.* 2009;151(1):28–36.

Linzer M, Visser MR, Oort FJ, Smets EM, McMurray JE, de Haes HC. Predicting and preventing physician burnout: results from the United States and the Netherlands. *Am J Med.* 2001;111(2):170–175.

Maslach C, Leiter M. *The Truth About Burnout: How Organizations Cause Personal Stress and What to Do About It.* San Francisco, CA: Jossey-Bass. 2000.

Perez HR, Beyrouty M, Bennett K, et al. Chaos in the clinic: characteristics and consequences of practices perceived as chaotic. *J Healthcare Qual.* 2015. Nov 12. [E-pub ahead of print].

Shanafelt TD. Physician burnout: stop blaming the individual.

Shanafelt TD, Gorringe G, Menaker R, et al. Impact of organizational leadership on physician burnout and satisfaction. *Mayo Clin Proc.* 2015;90(4):432–440.

Shanafelt TD, West CP, Sloan JA, et al. Career fit and burnout among academic faculty. *Arch Intern Med.* 2009;169(10):990–995.

Sinsky CA, Willard-Grace R, Schutzbank AM, Sinsky TA, Margolius D, Bodenheimer T. In search of joy in practice: a report of 23 high-functioning primary care practices. *Ann Fam Med.* 2013;11(3):272–278.

Ubel P. The joy has been sucked out of medicine. Here's why. [Blog]. 2015. Available at: http://www.kevinmd.com/blog/2015/11/the-joy-has-been-sucked-out-of-medicine-heres-why.html. Accessed May 24, 2016.

# CHAPTER 6

## THE IMPACT OF LEADERSHIP

*Leadership is the stewardship of the lives entrusted to you.*
—BOB CHAPMAN, AUTHOR OF *EVERYBODY MATTERS: THE EXTRAORDINARY POWER OF CARING FOR YOUR PEOPLE LIKE FAMILY*, PERSONAL COMMUNICATION, DECEMBER 17, 2015

*Management is doing things right; leadership is doing the right things.*
—PETER F. DRUCKER, MANAGEMENT CONSULTANT, EDUCATOR, AND AUTHOR [1]

O ver the course of our research for *Preventing Physician Burnout*, it became increasingly clear to us that the C-suite has a major role in physician burnout. In this chapter we will review leadership's impact on the drivers of burnout.

Health care leaders today face many difficult challenges. Peter F. Drucker, quoted above, also said, "Health care is the most difficult, chaotic, and complex industry to manage." (Drucker 2002) Each hospital is an amalgamation of many different operations and support services. Today's health care systems often include a number of hospitals as well as physician groups, home health agencies, and increasingly, insurance companies. Each of these entities has a different business model. It

---

1 Drucker PF. *Essential Drucker: The Best of Sixty Years of Peter Drucker's Essential Writings on Management.* New York: HarperCollins. 2001.

is impossible for any single leader to have competent expertise in all aspects of the business.

In addition to the complexity inherent in health care, organizational leaders are subject to intense pressures to

- ensure patient safety,
- achieve high quality,
- provide high levels of patient satisfaction,
- maintain a vibrant professional workforce,
- stay ahead of their competitors in providing the latest state-of-the-art technology,
- attract the highest quality physicians to their medical staff, and
- actively engage with leaders of other businesses and non-profits in their community—all while maintaining a financially healthy operation in a business with razor-thin profit margins.

It's no wonder that the turnover rate for hospital CEOs is the highest of any industry, with the tenure of a hospital CEO averaging about three years. CEOs constantly need to balance acting quickly and decisively in response to urgent business imperatives with taking the time to understand the root cause of an issue and lead a team through a collaborative approach to implementing the best possible strategy to address the problem.

Despite all these challenges, leaders are still ultimately responsible for the culture in their organization. The choices they make about what is important and how they lead their organizations to achieve have a greater impact on the organization's success than any other activity in the health care system.

How does this apply to physician burnout?

Burnout researchers have demonstrated a connection between destructive leadership behaviors and burnout. (Breevaart 2014) For example, abusive leadership, characterized by such behaviors as breaking promises or expressing anger at subordinates for things they did not do, is correlated with higher levels of emotional exhaustion. (Aryee 2008; Tepper 2000)

Recent research by Tait Shanafelt and colleagues at the Mayo Clinic has quantified the effect of leadership on physician burnout. (Shanafelt 2015) They found that a higher score of the department chair or division leader on 12 dimensions of leadership had a strong negative correlation with the burnout scores of individual physicians and a strong positive correlation with satisfaction. In fact, for each one-point increase in the overall leadership score, there was a 3 percent decrease in the likelihood of burnout. (Shanafelt 2015)

In addition, according to co-researchers Gene Beyt, MD, MS, physician and senior leadership coach at Interventional Learning Associates, and Richard M. Frankel, PhD, professor of medicine and research scientist at Indiana University School of Medicine and the Cleveland Clinic, too often leaders and boards are impatient to see immediate results from efforts at organizational culture change. Beyt and Frankel said, "Culture change is a marathon, not a sprint. It's more of an epic journey. You can reorganize a closet quickly, but creating a culture that does not burn out clinicians takes time."

We believe that top-down leadership is a primary root cause of the workplace stressors that are causing so many physicians to burn out. What do we mean by top-down leadership? What aspects of leadership style do we believe to be detrimental to the workplace? What are the characteristics of effective leadership? Our interviews with practicing physicians and leadership experts have clarified two key points: the enormity of the disconnect between physicians and leaders in many organizations and the existence of proven alternatives to traditional top-down leadership. We will describe some examples of these alternatives in Chapter 10. Key features of detrimental leadership styles include failure to manage external pressures, misaligned values, perceived lack of respect, and perceived lack of fairness.

Detrimental leadership styles persist in the health care environment for numerous reasons. Formal academic leadership programs often fail to provide sufficient training in interpersonal relationships and appreciation of the impact of relationships on staff resilience and burnout. Leaders-to-be are too often trained to play the role of ultimate decision-maker and too rarely develop the emotional intelligence needed to cultivate a collaborative, respectful culture or to motivate staff to reach their top potential. In addition, physicians are often promoted into positions of leadership based primarily on their clinical credentials—and are offered insufficient leadership training and mentoring to acquire these new skills and succeed as effective leaders.

## DISCONNECT FROM THE FRONT LINES

In most organizations there is a wide, and at times acrimonious, divide between physicians' professional goals and daily work experience and the administration's organizational goals and strategic priorities. Too often, leaders are unaware of the implications of their decisions on the experience of clinicians and on patient care. We believe this lack of awareness stems from a traditional view of the leader's role in health care and a lack of understanding that addressing the issues at the front lines of care will simultaneously reduce clinician burnout and improve organizational performance.

In our interviews and our review of online forums, we found that many physicians are distrustful of administrators. Some are downright angry. One obstetrician relayed a story about his previous employer, a hospital that had hired an expensive consulting company to address some workplace problems. "They paid thousands of dollars to hear what we had been saying all along. I think hiring that firm was to give us the illusion that administration cared. In the same way, meetings with administrators were to tell us what was decided, not to get our input." His bitterness about the administration's lack of understanding of the daily reality of clinicians ran deep. He told us, "Administrators want revenue and market share, and they don't care what it does to you. If we're stretched thin, they just don't care."

According to Beyt and Frankel, the problem partially stems from administrators and clinicians viewing each other as opposing camps. "Part of the issue is that we humans tend to 'other' each other. Some CEOs say, 'I don't get it. Why are physicians so difficult to engage?' To them we would reply, 'You get it by investing in relationships, being vulnerable, talking about what's meaningful to you, and listening to what's meaningful to physicians. That means changing the rules of engagement.'"

Robert Altman, MD, chair of obstetrics and gynecology at Sutter Gould Medical Foundation, also identified the failure of leaders to address problems as a key factor in physician burnout: "What can make the work situation worse is if you're working on problems every day and they never get fixed. It's like the experiments with dogs on an electrified floor. Initially they move to try to find a place that's not electrified, but when they figure out the whole floor is electrified, they don't bother moving. When you have problems day after day after day, that's when you get burnout."

Stephen Swensen, MD, medical director for leadership and organizational development at the Mayo Clinic, emphasized the importance of the leaders' connections to the front lines, saying, "Ninety-five percent of hospitals are led by administrators who haven't practiced medicine." The Mayo Clinic has developed a robust physician leadership development program. Swensen points to the program as a key reason that the burnout rate at the organization is about half the national average.

Although a thorough analysis of the roots of the divide between administration and physicians today is beyond the scope of this book, we want to highlight four primary causes for the disconnect: failure to effectively manage the effects of external pressures, misaligned values, perceived lack of respect, and perceived lack of fairness.

## FAILURE TO MANAGE EXTERNAL PRESSURES
In Paul's work as an executive coach and consultant, he sees CEOs who are confronted by increasingly potent external pressures demanding top levels of performance across all domains. They often react by increasing the performance expectations of physicians without fixing workplace issues that slow down efficiency and present barriers to quality care. When a CEO is faced with an imperative to reduce costs due to budget deficits or to improve financial performance in anticipation of an acquisition or bond issuance, they often reduce support staff and other resources that physicians view as necessary. James Womack of the Lean Enterprise Institute has seen this tendency as well. In an interview, he phrased it this way: "As more MBAs are involved in health care, they

focus first on finances. The result is that staff works harder and feels pushed. This is a considerable factor in burnout." Kristine Olsen, MD, MS, a health services researcher and assistant professor of clinical medicine at Yale School of Medicine, pointed to a lack of awareness of the intricacies of medical decision making as a cause of the failure to manage external pressures: "Non-clinical business people have some blind spots about the complexity of health care and most aren't aware of their blind spots."

Much depends on how we define success. Organizational leaders ask a lot of their physicians when they define success as seeing a higher volume of patients with more complex conditions while performing at ever-higher levels of quality, safety, patient satisfaction, and financial stewardship (read, "doing more with less"). Paul has consulted with several organizations whose executive leadership has set expectations of 75th to 90th percentile performance on key performance metrics while providing support staff at 10th to 25th percentile levels. It is possible to do so, but not without heroic efforts on the part of frontline clinicians, which is simply unsustainable in the long run. Such heroics negatively affect the physician's work performance and other aspects of his or her life. They require sacrificing time for family, friends, or personal care. (It *is* possible to achieve these outcomes without such sacrifice in an organization that has a mature Lean management system and culture.)

## MISALIGNED VALUES

The leader sets the culture first through developing and communicating the vision, mission, and values of the organization. Vision and mission statements are common in all health care organizations. They are usually based on the organization's values.

The real power of vision, mission, and values statements comes from the way the organization develops, communicates, and exemplifies these guiding documents. A collaborative process that involves all stakeholders achieves a significantly different result than a process involving only the top leaders of the organization.

Physicians place a high value on providing the best quality care possible to their patients. All health care organizations include quality care as one of their values. As previously noted, when a leader acts in a way that physicians perceive as contrary to the value of providing high-quality care, a burned-out physician is quick to cynically point this out to anyone who will listen.

Peter Anderson, MD, founder of Team Care Medicine, sees this conflict play out across the country in what he describes as a huge chasm between administration and clinical doctors. "Administrators refuse to provide more staff to physicians when they are experiencing losses of $80,000 per primary care physician. Physicians are unwilling to change their practice styles to address financial viability issues." The key stake holders are under such stress that they are unable to focus on common core values such as ensuring sustainable, high-quality care for their communities.

## PERCEIVED LACK OF RESPECT

Physicians consider themselves to be the professional equals of hospital CEOs and are highly sensitive to administrative actions that may impact their ability to provide high-quality care. When leaders reduce expenses by cutting back on staff, physicians recognize that the decision has a greater impact on their daily work experience than on that of the leaders. The staffing cuts exacerbate the drivers of physician burnout, namely, the intensity, time demand, and complexity of the work.

Many physicians perceive, rightly or wrongly, that the number of administrators in corporate offices continues to grow while the number of people working on the front lines of patient care decreases. Even if the frontline staffing numbers remain constant, replacing experienced, knowledgeable staff with employees whose licensing, skill sets, and experience level are not the same can exacerbate the chaos and perceived stress in the workplace.

Actions such as these reinforce physicians' perception that the administration does not share their values or care about their ability to provide the highest quality care. Some leaders minimize the risk of such negative perceptions by

- involving physicians in developing the vision, mission, and values statements;
- communicating the rationale for decisions that may adversely impact physicians; and
- connecting personally with physicians and meeting with them on their home turf of the doctors' lounge, dining room, or hospital wards.

In the absence of such efforts to collaborate, physicians understandably interpret the administration's actions as displaying a lack of respect. As we have discussed previously, Kerry Patterson and his co-authors wrote, "Respect is like air; if you take it away, it's all people can think about." (Patterson 2012) Respect is essential for effective working relationships between physicians and leadership.

In our interview with John Toussaint, he echoed these sentiments: "The biggest impact on the physician's life is the management of the organization where they work. This will define whether they are stressed out or not. Management activities are the root cause of most burn-out for health care providers. If you have a crappy manager with top-down, Sloan-style management, it will make your life miserable." Craig Albanese of New York-Presbyterian/Morgan Stanley Children's Hospital and Sloane Hospital for Women emphasized the importance of regular communication from leaders. Without it, according to Albanese, physicians tend to fill in the gap with negative perceptions of leadership, thinking that administration neither knows nor cares about their problems. Albanese told us, "The paranoia, the defeatist attitude comes from not enough information, and it feeds burnout."

## PERCEIVED LACK OF FAIRNESS

In the current health care environment, with multiple competing demands and thin financial margins that limit resource availability, leaders face significant challenges when making decisions about the allocation of limited resources. Given these challenges, it's not surprising that some physicians will see the decisions as unfair. We will present three scenarios in which physicians may perceive a lack of fairness on the part of leadership.

## MARKETING PROMISES THAT EXCEED OPERATIONAL CAPACITY

Health care systems are under intense pressure to increase their market share, especially for services that are well reimbursed and therefore support the bottom line. One way to increase the market share of such services is by adding or enhancing high-end specialty service lines such as cardiovascular medicine, sports medicine, and cancer care. Success depends not only on the effective development and operation of the program but also on an effective marketing campaign. In an interview, a director of patient experience at a major teaching center described how the marketing program for a new center of excellence was developed concurrently with operational development, yet the care providers did not feel ready to deliver on the marketing promise when the campaign went public. In such cases, physicians often feel that they are unfairly expected to deliver on a promise the health system has made to their patients.

## DIVERSION OF THE LEADER'S FOCUS TO MERGERS AND ACQUISITIONS

Another approach to gaining market power is growth through merger or acquisition. In the highly regulated world of health care, mergers and acquisitions are complex transactions that have far-reaching implications. They place significant demands on leaders' time–time that could be spent otherwise connecting with frontline care providers. As we have discussed, patient care processes on the front lines are often dysfunctional or chaotic. Care providers often feel they are struggling to get through the day without injuring a patient. When physicians see the administrators spending more time trying to add another dysfunctional hospital to their already frustrating work environment, they perceive that the leadership has their priorities misplaced and deem that to be unfair.

## COST ALLOCATIONS FOR HIGH-COST ITEMS

Another common fairness issue is the process of allocating capital expenditures on high-cost items that the health system purchases to support diagnostic and interventional treatment procedures. Every system has a finite amount of funds available to spend on big-ticket requests. Different specialties compete for approval to purchase high-tech equipment that will allow them to provide the latest state-of-the-art care to their patients. The availability of the newest equipment is advantageous for the physician; often procedures that use the equipment receive a higher reimbursement rate. In addition, the physician reaps the reward of new patients who will seek out the most up-to-date medical care.

This challenge brings to light two fairness issues. The first issue is whether providing care with the newest technology is truly in the interest of the system and the patient. In many cases the additional clinical benefits are marginal, whereas the additional expense is substantial for the system and the patient. Physicians and others may question whether another use of the funds would have better served patients, the system, and the community.

The second fairness issue relates to the process for selecting the items in which the system will invest. These items incur large expenses, which has significant implications for clinical care and financial performance. As such, the CEO and CFO often feel compelled to control the selection process. However, when they do, the physicians whose requested expenditures were not selected will naturally feel that they have been treated unfairly. Some CEOs take a different approach. They assign a group of physician stakeholders who represent all the key interests to choose how the capital budget will be allocated within parameters that the CEO and the physicians agree on. This process requires more work, as the physician representatives of each stakeholder need to learn the relative costs and benefits not only of the choice for which they are advocating but also of the choices of the other specialties. This process of empowerment and mutual decision making significantly reduces the perception of unfairness in the capital budget allocation process.

∫∫∫

One key role of a health care leader is to support the frontline clinicians as they pursue the work of caring for patients. When physicians perceive that their leaders are not committed to helping them by providing needed support, they become frustrated. When leaders perceive that the physicians are pursuing their own self-interest over the interests of the patient, they find it hard to support such physicians. We believe there is a better way. Lean Done Right, based deeply in the principle of Respect for People, offers a framework that builds respect and collaboration into the management approach. We will discuss this further in Chapter 11.

## REFERENCES

Aryee S, Sun LY, Chen ZXG, Debrah YA. Abusive supervision and contextual performance: the mediating role of emotional exhaustion and the moderating role of work unit structure. *Manag Org Rev.* 2008;4:393–411.

Breevaart K, Bakker AB, Hetland J, Hetland H. The influence of constructive and destructive leadership behaviors on follower burnout. In: Leiter MP, Bakker AB, Maslach C, eds. *Burnout at Work: A Psychological Perspective.* New York: Psychological Press. 2014:102–121.

Drucker P. *Managing in the Next Society.* New York: Truman Talley Books. 2002.

Patterson K, Grenny J. McMillan R, Switzler A. *Crucial Conversations: Tools for Talking When Stakes Are High.* New York: McGraw-Hill. 2012.

Shanafelt TD, Gorringe G, Menaker R, Storz KA, Reeves D, Buskirk SJ, et al. Impact of organizational leadership on physician burnout and satisfaction. *Mayo Clin Proc.* 2015;90(4):432–440.

Tepper BJ. Is there a relationship between burnout and objective performance? A critical review of 16 studies. *Work Stress.* 2000;43:178–190.

# CHAPTER 7
## THE IMPACT OF THE EHR ON THE WORKPLACE

*Electronic health records hold great promise for enhancing coordination of care and improving quality of care. In their current form and implementation, however, they have had a number of unintended negative consequences including reducing efficiency, increasing clerical burden, and increasing the risk of burnout for physicians.*
—TAIT SHANAFELT, MD, DIRECTOR, MAYO CLINIC DEPARTMENT PROGRAM ON PHYSICIAN WELL-BEING [1]

*With our new EHR, the processes were so cumbersome that overnight seeing 10 patients felt like seeing 20.*
—DAVID BUTLER, MD, VICE PRESIDENT OF EHR TRANSFORMATION AND OPTIMIZATION FOR SUTTER HEALTH, PERSONAL COMMUNICATION, FEBRUARY 18, 2016

I nnovation has had a significant impact on many service industries. We no longer enter a bank to manage financial transactions. We make our travel arrangements online. With a few taps on our phone, we can call for a ride, find nearby restaurants, read reviews, and make reservations or order a meal. We track our activity level with a digital

---

1 Mayo Clinic. Electronic medical practice environment can lead to physician burnout. [Internet]. June 27, 2016. Available at: http://newsnetwork.mayoclinic.org/discussion/electronic-medical-practice-environment-can-lead-to-physician-burnout/. Accessed September 2, 2016.

device. It is increasingly common to think of a service need and ask, "Is there an app for that?"

The EHR represents one of the most significant examples of a disruptive innovation catalyzing a sweeping change across an industry. A majority of hospitals and physician practices now have a patient portal into the EHR where patients can send messages, check lab results, make appointments, and pay their bills. (DHHS 2014) However, innovations like these are relatively new to health care.

Given the way digitization has revolutionized other service industries, many experts and clinicians have held high expectations for what computerization, and specifically the EHR, can do for health care, including:

- The ability to collect and analyze large amounts of data, which is necessary for delivering on population health
- Increased efficiency, given the ability to communicate quickly with multiple caregivers
- Cost savings, with the reduction of duplicate testing, for example
- Reduced medical errors, with better identification of potential drug interactions and the virtual elimination of handwriting mistakes
- The ability to use artificial intelligence to aid diagnostic accuracy and treatment effectiveness
- The ability to provide personalized precision medicine

Ronald A. Paulus, MD, president and CEO of Mission Health, a large, integrated health system headquartered in Asheville, North Carolina, described the balance of advantages and disadvantages of the EHR this way: "The EHR is neither an angel or a devil. It's both. There's no question that EHRs are needed to improve population health, and many safety improvements are impossible without an the EHR. Everyone forgets that before we had EHRs, nobody had any real idea what drugs someone was on, never reconciled meds substantively, no one could tell who was a diabetic in their practice. We tend to take all those benefits for granted and focus on what we don't like."

These are definite advantages of the EHR that benefit both care providers and patients. However, "upgrading" information systems in health care is especially challenging because of the high complexity and high degree of risk associated with health care delivery.

## THE CHALLENGE OF DIGITALIZATION IN HEALTH CARE

More than other industries, health care involves significant complexity in the variation of problems encountered, skill sets of stakeholders, types of interfacing devices and software systems, and workflow processes. Layered on this complexity are the multiple risks inherent in the field. In health care, there is little room for error. Operations cannot be fully shut down for repairs or upgrades. There is exposure due to malpractice as well as to billing and compliance regulations. Organizations are privy to large volumes of personal information for which loss or theft will incur substantial penalties. And most health care organizations run on a thin operating margin that limits the financial resources available to help deal with the disruption and change associated with the EHR adoption.

In addition to the anticipated challenges of digitalization, there have also been a number of unintended consequences that have had a drastic impact on physicians and other clinicians.

## THE UNINTENDED CONSEQUENCES OF THE EHR

Although the EHR solves many problems of the pre-digital age, it has also created many new problems. These primarily include an uptick in the time devoted to non-clinical tasks, less efficient workflow, negative effects on interpersonal relationships, and negative effects on the quality of care.

**Increased Time Devoted to Non-clinical Tasks.** The advent of EHR has translated into a shift in how clinicians spend their days. For many, the EHR has meant more time spent on non-clinical tasks, which has had several secondary effects. First, the increase in time spent on such tasks is inconsistent with the career goals of physicians and is a source of frustration. Data entry does not exemplify a highly trained clinician working at the top of his or her license.

As Robert Wachter at University of California, San Francisco, put it, "The EHR is an underemphasized joy zapper. Here you are doing what you are most trained fundamentally to do—talk with a patient and establish an emotional bond with them—and instead you are doing this thing that is essentially secretarial work. Not only is it a distraction from what you think you could and should be doing, but it's created a vibe in the office, so the patient begins to believe you don't care. It is so ultimately destructive of purpose and joy that until we fix that, it is hard to figure out how physicians could bring back the joy and passion they came into the profession to have."

Second, the time spent on non-clinical tasks steals time away from clinical responsibilities. With today's fiscal pressures, physicians are under pressure to recoup this lost revenue. The funneling of clerical work toward clinicians represents a wasted use of resources, which would probably not be tolerated in other industries. As Christine Sinsky, MD, of the American Medical Association, wrote with co-authors in a 2006 report for the Society for General Internal Medicine, "In few other sectors of the economy is the highest level professional responsible for the majority of production, customer service, and clerical work." (Babbott 2006) A recent study for which Sinsky was the principal investigator found that physicians working in ambulatory sites spent almost 50 percent of their total time on clerical work and EHR but only 27 percent on direct clinical time with patients. (Sinsky 2016) In effect, physicians are spending two hours on the computer for every one hour in direct patient care. In addition, the physicians who completed a time diary reported spending one to two hours each evening on additional EHR-related work. Sinsky and others have called the effect of the EHR on interactions with patients "distracted doctoring," and likened it to operating a motor vehicle while texting. [Sinsky 2013] They point out that although the EHR can be considered an intrinsic component of patient care—unlike texting while driving—the multitasking involved in data entry can distract the care provider from the core activities of the patient encounter.

Third, the increase in non-clinical work has a profound effect on the work-life balance of physicians. Many of the physicians we interviewed described the spillover effect on their personal lives. They describe spending more time working in their "off hours," at home on evenings and weekends, because of the increased data-entry demands as well as the ability to work anytime at any location. In the early 2000s, Paul had the personal experience, as a family physician participating in an the EHR go-live at a nationally known health system, of falling asleep at the keyboard in his home office on several occasions while trying to finish up progress notes and respond to inbox notices from the day's work.

Fourth, the increase in clerical tasks has translated into more time spent on a keyboard. As a result, more physicians are experiencing work-related injuries, such as repetitive-use injury. Paul recently learned that 10 of the 11 ophthalmologists at a large health system in California have some degree of repetitive-strain syndrome in their hands. These injuries are especially concerning for physicians who routinely perform delicate, high-stakes procedures.

**Less Efficient Workflow.** The EHR may eventually streamline and support efficient workflows in clinical settings. To date, however, it has impeded efficiency in many organizations. In many instances, inefficient, non-intuitive design and lack of communication with other systems have made the EHR a major impediment to efficient workflow. In the course of Paul's work, he has witnessed the scope of this inefficiency. By his estimation, physician productivity, measured by the number of patients seen per day, has dropped by 20 to 40 percent with the advent of the EHR. According to an online article, a 2013 research consulting firm found that 66 percent of physicians surveyed reported a drop in productivity, measured as patients seen per day, after implementation of the EHR. (Millard 2013)

**Negative Effects on Interpersonal Relationships.** The EHR has had a tremendous negative impact on interpersonal relationships. Physicians and nurses now spend less time directly interacting with patients and with each other. In-person interactions have been replaced by electronic communication. When there was a single hard copy of the patient's record, a physician would go to the chart to review or enter new information, thus interacting with nurses, staff, and other physicians. With the EHR, there is a universally available electronic copy of the chart, obviating the need to communicate face-to-face with colleagues.

As Wachter describes in *The Digital Doctor: Hope, Hype, and Harm at the Dawn of Medicine's Computer Age*, this shift has had a profound effect on a physician's work life. (Wachter 2015)

> Prior to digitization of X-rays, the radiology department in most hospitals was a hub of activity every morning as attending physicians would come down (imaging is almost universally in the basement or on the ground floor) to review their patient's X-rays and other imaging studies with the radiologists...The radiologists knew almost all attending physicians personally and were tuned into much of what was happening in the hospital. Nowadays, attending physicians review the images and the radiologists' reports from anywhere but the imaging department. They rarely meet face-to-face with the radiologist. The radiologist job has changed dramatically, as they now grind through reading images at an ever faster pace with minimal interaction with other physicians.

The adoption of the EHR has also negatively affected physicians' relationship with their patients. Physicians spend more time looking at the computer screen and less time eye-to-eye with their patients. Patient satisfaction has declined, in part because physicians often face the computer screen to enter data during the visit rather than face the patient. (Friedberg 2015) The need to document information in the medical record—and do so as efficiently as possible—has compromised personal contact and nonverbal communication.

**Negative Effects on the Quality of Care.** Although the EHR holds the potential to reduce a number of different types of medical errors that adversely affect patient safety, some types of errors are more likely with the EHR. (Garber 2014; Maryland Hospital Patient Safety Program 2014) Poorly designed software can lead to mistakes in ordering tests and treatments, which can increase the risk to patients and increase the ultimate expense of care. In his book, Wachter describes one such error in which a child hospitalized at a highly respected academic medical center received an antibiotic dose 38.5 times that intended, primarily because of the complex, user-unfriendly interface for ordering medications. (Wachter 2015)

The EHR has also had some negative effects on the quality of communication and on patient records. To save time, many clinicians cut and paste information within the record template, potentially introducing errors. In addition, the structured fields of the EHR favor consistency, but at the expense of the individuality of clinicians' notes. Many physicians we interviewed described the disadvantages of the "generic note." They lamented that progress notes have lost their value as a means to communicate patient-specific diagnostic considerations and treatment plans between clinicians.

## THE ROLE OF REGULATIONS

The Meaningful Use initiative has catalyzed the adoption of EHRs across the country. However, the regulations related to the program have caused issues that adversely affect clinicians.

According to David K. Butler at Sutter Health, one important effect has been a reduction in the quality of clinical information. "Some critical thinking gets lost. The admitting physician needs to put all the orders in the computer at once and all orders are considered equally important—a life-saving medication and a small diet change are treated the same in the EHR. Some physicians feel they need to ask every single question on the admission page, even if they are inappropriate for the situation."

An unintended consequence of the regulations is confusion about which members of the clinical team—the physician, advanced practice provider, registered nurse, licensed practical nurse, or medical assistant—are permitted to enter information into the chart. Many organizations have interpreted the regulations conservatively and, due to concerns about being able to bill for an encounter, have required physicians to enter certain information. However, as Steven Mitnick, MD, chief medical officer of the Sutter Gould Medical Foundation, told us, these interpretations are not always substantiated by the regulations. Frustration with EHRs in general and with the Meaningful Use regulations in particular, has led some physicians to give it the moniker "Meaningless Abuse."

## WHAT WENT WRONG WITH THE EHR?

We believe the gap between the anticipated benefits of EHRs and the current reality results from several oversights, many of which reflect a failure to appreciate the complexity of health care.

### Failure to fix broken processes before digitalization

In an attempt to save money and time implementing EHRs, most organizations did not redesign and optimize their clinical workflows prior to adoption of the computerized systems; instead, they superimposed the new technology onto established inefficient processes. On a larger scale, the national health care system was not redesigned prior to the widespread push for electronic communication and documentation. As Wachter told us, "I think the issues with EHRs have more to do with the fundamental economics of health care and the need for a deep reboot of how we organize everything." James Hereford of Stanford University Medical Center voiced a similar sentiment, saying, "We did not improve the workflow processes before moving to the EHR, so instead of being an enabler, it's a veneer on top of a broken system. Other industries addressed the underlying work processes 25 years ago."

### Failure to ensure clinician-oriented, user-friendly design

Most EHR systems are designed to optimize charge capture rather than to facilitate communication among care providers and documentation of patient care. Navigating through the patient record is not easy or intuitive. Butler shared an insight he had one winter a few years ago. He had been struggling with the newly implemented EHR at work, as he cared for a patient in the ICU. He arrived home to find his ten-year-old son easily navigating the computer game he'd received just a few hours earlier. "My son was playing a complicated computer game with lots of options, interacting with other players from across the country, while at the hospital, where patients' lives are at stake, I couldn't figure out how to place the order for a patient on a dopamine drip. It's a question of poor usability."

## Failure to dedicate sufficient IT support staff

Too often, organizations fail to dedicate sufficient information technology (IT) support staff to facilitate implementation and ongoing use of the EHR. Because most IT departments do not have the staff to meet the work demands, the queue of requests for fixes or upgrades is long, making it difficult to respond quickly to urgent requests. For this and other reasons, clinicians at the front lines often find themselves without the assistance they need to identify and fix the problems they encounter. They often resort to work-arounds to complete their work and submit requests for aid only after they have tried all other options, are in urgent need of help, and are utterly frustrated with the barriers to efficient patient care.

In addition, the relationship between the IT department and clinical units is often problematic. In most industries, the IT department is a support function that focuses on serving the frontline worker. In health care, too often the IT department sees itself as an entity that must meet service-level metrics, the most prominent being to keep within its budget. For example, often the chief information officer (CIO) reports directly to the CEO and enjoys a status that is equal to or greater than that of the chief operating officer or chief medical officer. This organizational structure creates a system in which the requests of end users for support are often met with resistance or fall through the cracks in the organization's bureaucracy.

## Failure to design systems with human factors in mind

Too often, EHR systems are not designed to take into account the fact that users are human—and prone to human error. For example, the alerts in poorly designed systems signal so frequently that physicians often click through them without fully evaluating the warnings. If systems were designed with human factors in mind, the frequency of warnings would have been identified as a problem before implementation. Earlier in this chapter we described a case from Wachter's book in which a child at an academic medical center received an antibiotic dose 38.5 times that intended. The event resulted from multiple errors, one of which was the fact that the pediatric resident ignored the alarms in the CPOE about the prescribed dose. Her behavior was in keeping with a lesson from the "hidden curriculum" passed from one trainee to another to ignore the signals. Why? Because there were so many, and "she knew that doing so was the only way she could get her work done." (Wachter 2015)

### Failure to ensure interoperability

EHR vendors have guarded their territory carefully and have not made interoperability between systems a priority. The failure of regulatory bodies to insist on reliable, easy communication between the various EHR systems has made the safety of patient care more difficult to ensure and has inserted additional barriers and frustrations into the delivery of care.

As described in a 2014 RAND study, the 2009 American Recovery and Reinvestment Act included a major section related to health care—Health Information Technology for Economic and Clinical Health (HITECH). (Garber 2014) The intent of HITECH regulations was to improve EHR usability and interoperability. However, the Health and Human Services guide to EHR implementation prioritized health care providers' rapid implementation of existing EHR products over improved usability and interoperability. The intended benefits of HITECH have not yet been realized, and the result for physicians is increased clerical burden and daily frustrations.

More recent legislation aims to address these issues, however. Under the Medicare Access and CHIP Reauthorization Act of 2015 (MACRA), interoperability is defined as the ability for two or more disparate health technologies to exchange clinical information and to use that information under a standard set of guidelines to coordinate patient care, ultimately improving patient outcomes. (Department of Health and Human Services 2016) Currently, the Department of Health and Human Services is drafting a set of metrics to measure interoperability relative to this definition and determine whether the stated goal of "widespread interoperability" is successfully met by December 31, 2018. (HIMSS 2016)

### Failure to anticipate the impact on clinicians

A major flaw in the widespread implementation of EHR was the failure to carefully consider the downstream effects on clinicians. For a number of reasons, physicians have borne much of the "squeeze" associated with the digitalization of health care. The electronic systems "allow" others to ask or require that physicians perform more data entry. As Wachter put it, "The EHR enables people to ask physicians to do just a bit more here and a bit more there for documentation. But it all adds up." Sinsky agreed, telling us, "The EHR was not designed for advanced care. For this reason, it pushes more work to the physician."

Wachter also emphasized the increase in patients' electronic access to physicians as a workload issue that has not been clearly addressed. "The EHR enables patient access to physicians 24/7. Mostly this is good, but no thought was given to how this work is paid for or to the change in the physician's job description." At Paul's previous organization, Sutter Gould Medical Foundation, a study showed that for every patient seen in the office, a physician would receive non-visit-related, inbox activities for another four patients, including PPO authorizations, formulary requests, and documentation for Medicare, nursing homes, and home health facilities.

Many physicians feel pressured because of the time needed to manage electronic communication that is related to patient care or that involves direct communication with patients. Because these tasks are rarely compensated, physicians must find time to complete them in addition to their other responsibilities. Many physicians also see the extra unpaid work as a fairness issue.

### Failure to anticipate the impact on interpersonal relationships

An important oversight in widespread EHRs adoption was the failure to consider the effects on the relationship between the physician and his or her patient and the relationship of clinicians with each other. As we've discussed, the insertion of the computer screen into the patient encounter often has negative effects for both patient and physician. In his book, Wachter makes the case that the introduction of computers into health care has fundamentally changed patient care and relationships among care providers and between care providers and patients. (Wachter 2015) The increased time that clinicians spend communicating via devices instead of face-to-face affects their sense of camaraderie and represents an erosion of community, which Maslach and Leiter found to be a key driver of workplace burnout. (Maslach 2008)

## THE IMPACT OF THE EHR ON PHYSICIANS

Many physicians have a love-hate relationship with the EHR. They *love* accessing readily available information in the EHR. They love the ability to quickly pull up old records, test results, imaging studies, and current medical literature and the ability to analyze data from an individual patient or a population of patients in charts and graphs. They *hate* the process of inputting new data, which is time intensive and reduces many physicians to data entry clerks for a significant part of their day. They are frustrated by the inefficient design of many the EHR systems, which are better suited for coding and billing than for clinical care.

A 2013 RAND study for the AMA found that physicians generally support EHRs in concept. (Friedman 2013) However, multiple issues with the daily use of EHRs adversely affect physicians' job satisfaction. The constellation of non-intuitive interfaces, additional time spent on lower-level skills, interference with the relationship with patients, and other frustrating, potentially risky, and burdensome aspects of EHRs have made them a lightning rod for physician discontent and job frustration. The burden imposed by the EHR is a flash point for many physicians. Online forums are rife with the condemnation of the EHR as a major source of dissatisfaction among doctors. As Craig Albanese of New York-Presbyterian/Morgan Stanley Children's Hospital and Sloane Hospital for Women told us, "EHR is killing health care. Our new the EHR is a wonderful cost accounting system, but is terrible for workflows. We are in the clinic till 7:00 or 8:00 p.m., or we take work home."

Sinsky has found the EHR to be a common complaint in her interviews with physicians across the country: "Physicians tell me that this technology makes it hard to provide eye contact and full, undivided attention when interacting with the patient. Plus, some of the Meaningful Use requirements are cumbersome. We cannot give the patient the handout and then record that we did and have it count for Meaningful Use. Instead, the computer must prompt us to give the handout, and the handout must come from the EHR to count."

In our interview, Wachter pointed out that in the short term, the EHR has vastly increased physicians' workload and the time pressure they experience and has significantly interfered with the source of meaning in their work: direct interactions with patients.

Research substantiates physicians' personal belief that the EHR factors into the increase in physician burnout. A 2016 nationwide study from the Mayo Clinic documented that physicians who used the EHR with computerized physician order entry (CPOE) were at higher risk for burnout—whether or not they reported being dissatisfied with the system they used. (Shanafelt 2016) The researchers calculated that physicians using CPOE had about a 30 percent higher risk of burnout than those who did not. Physicians who used an EHR (with or without CPOE) were less satisfied with the amount of time they spent on clerical tasks than physicians who did not use an EHR, regardless of age, sex, specialty, practice setting, or hours worked per week. Interestingly, of the physicians who used an EHR, less than four in ten agreed that the EHR had improved patient care (36 percent agreed; 41 percent disagreed).

As Wachter told us, "Computers transform our relationships and our workflow. For docs, the EHR is one of the main contributors to burnout."

## TECHNOLOGY BEYOND THE EHR

The EHR is not the sole innovation in information technology affecting health care. The use of telehealth has also expanded. Physicians can treat patients for simple, acute problems via a video visit. Many doctors have signed up with services providing video visits, often working in their off hours for additional pay, although the fee is smaller than that for in-person visits. Some experts are concerned about the quality of care delivered and the impact of video visits on continuity of care. (Huff 2014) However, telehealth saves a substantial amount of time for patients in rural areas, who would otherwise need to drive several hours for visits that might be just a few minutes in duration.

And more changes loom on the horizon. EHRs generate enormous amounts of data, as do monitoring devices in hospitals and increasingly popular wearable devices. The growing ability to analyze this "big data" provides various stakeholders with valuable information, which will allow:

- Patients to better understand how their behaviors impact their health
- Physicians to better understand their patients' health habits, adherence with treatment plans, and risk factors
- Health systems to better understand and compare physician practice patterns, quality, and cost effectiveness, as well as the revenue and expense drivers of their financial performance
- Employers and payers to better understand and compare health system performance

The increasing automation of the analysis of big data will bring unprecedented change to health care delivery. Such analysis has the potential to help improve the health of populations and add to our understanding of risk factors and prevention strategies through research. However, it also has the potential to add complexity to care delivery, flood each patient's chart with data that may or may not be relevant, and increase liability exposure for physicians who miss an early warning sign of a potentially serious diagnosis (even if missing the early sign would not change the course of disease or prognosis)—all of which will further increase physicians' stress and the risk of burnout.

∫∫∫

We believe the lion's share of the negative consequences seen with widespread EHR adoption—including the uptick in burnout among physicians—stems from poor software design and the implementation of the

EHR into the workplace without first redesigning dysfunctional work processes. These underlying problems can be solved by working with frontline providers at the point of care to redesign clinical workflows to maximize the value of the EHR and to avoid undue stress on clinicians. Both the design of EHR systems and the design of clinical workflows must be fixed to solve the problems related to EHRs.

Improved design of EHR systems is beyond the scope of this book, although in Chapter 12 we will touch on specific strategies that organizations can use to ensure improved usability and to advocate for better interoperability. We will discuss clinical workflow solutions in Part 3.

In the next chapter, we'll describe the external drivers—those outside the organization—that are exerting unprecedented pressure on health care organizations and on the physicians who work within them.

## REFERENCES

Babbott SF, Bigby JA, Day SC, et al. Redesigning the practice model for general internal medicine: a proposal for coordinated care. A policy monograph. Society for General Internal Medicine. 2006. Available at: http://impak.sgim.org/userfiles/file/SGIMReports/ BRPFinalReport71106.pdf. Accessed July 4, 2016.

Department of Health and Human Services. The Office of the National Coordinator for Health Information Technology. Interoperability measurement for the MACRA section 106(b). 2016. Available at: https:// www.healthit.gov/FACAS/sites/faca/files/HITJC_Interoperability_ MACRA_RFI_Briefing_Presentation_04-19-16.pdf. Accessed September 27, 2016.

Department of Health and Human Services. The Office of the National Coordinator for Health Information Technology. US hospital adoption of patient engagement functionalities. 2014. Available at: http:// dashboard.healthit.gov/quickstats/pages/FIG-Hospital-Adoption-of-Patient-Engagement-Functionalities.php. Accessed July 8, 2016.

Friedberg MW, Chen PG, Van Busum KR, et al. Factors affecting physician professional satisfaction and their implications for patient care, health systems, and health policy. RAND Corporation. 2013.

Available at: http://www.rand.org/pubs/research_reports/RR439. html. Accessed May 12, 2016.

Garber S, Gates SM, Keeler EB, et al. Research report: redirecting innovation in US health care: options to decrease spending and increase value: case studies. RAND Corporation. 2014. Available at: http://www.rand.org/pubs/research_reports/RR308.html. Accessed July 8, 2016.

HIMSS Electronic Health Record Association. Interoperability in healthcare fact sheet. June 2016. Available at: http://www.himssehra. org/docs/InteropStatus_FactSheet_Final_Links.pdf. Accessed September 26, 2016.

Huff C. Virtual visits pose real issues for physicians. ACP Internist. 2014. American College of Physicians. Available at: http://www.acpinternist.org/archives/2014/11/virtual-visit.htm. Accessed July 8, 2016.

Maryland Hospital Patient Safety Program. Annual report: fiscal year 2013. 2014. Available at: http://dhmh.maryland.gov/ohcq/HOS/Docs/Reports/Hospital%20Patient%20Safety%20Report,%20FY13,%20FINAL.pdf. Accessed July 8, 2016.

Maslach C, Leiter MP. Early predictors of job burnout and engagement. J Appl Psychol. 2008;93(3):498–512.

Millard M. Docs blame EHRs for lost productivity. 2013. Available at: http://www.healthcareitnews.com/news/docs-blame-ehrs-lost-productivity. Accessed July 8, 2016.

Shanafelt TD, Dyrbye LN, Sinsky C, et al. Relationship between clerical burden and characteristics of the electronic environment with physician burnout and professional satisfaction. Mayo Clin Proc. 2016. Jun 10. [E-pub ahead of print].

Sinsky C, Colligan L, Li L, et al. Allocation of physician time in ambulatory practice: a time and motion study in 4 specialties. Ann Intern Med. 2016. Sept 6. [E-pub ahead of print.]

Sinsky CA, Beasley JW. Texting While Doctoring: A Patient Safety Hazard. Ann Intern Med. 2013;159:782–783.

Wachter R. The Digital Doctor: Hope, Hype, and Harm at the Dawn of Medicine's Computer Age. New York: McGraw-Hill. 2015:127–142.

# CHAPTER 8

## EXTERNAL DRIVERS

*The increased volume of care for acutely ill and complex patients requires time that many docs just don't have.*
—WAYNE SOTILE, PHD, FOUNDER, CENTER FOR PHYSICIAN RESILIENCE

*So much is driven from outside, the external environment. And every year it gets worse. We have to run faster to stay in the same place.*
—STEVEN MITNICK, MD, CHIEF MEDICAL OFFICER, SUTTER GOULD MEDICAL FOUNDATION

Health care is, by its nature, a very complex operational environment.

- **It is capital- and labor-intensive.** Individuals working on the front lines of patient care are some of the most highly educated people in the world. They use some of the most advanced—and expensive—technology in the workforce.
- **It is constantly changing.** New technological innovations are introduced daily. There is a constant deluge of new medical knowledge, making it virtually impossible for clinicians to keep current on new diagnostic and treatment options. Reimbursement for most services is decreasing, while the costs of doing business are

increasing. Medical records have quickly moved from paper to computers.

- *Patient care is demanding, rife with requirements, and highly litigious.* Health care providers deal with life and death on a daily basis. The stakes are high to get things right. Required documentation can steal time away from activities that are important to providing good care.

As James Hereford of Stanford Health told us, "Health care is complex. It's capital-intensive and labor-intensive. It is a knowledge-management business with very highly educated frontline workers. Plus, it's a very challenging service environment, because you are dealing with people at their most vulnerable." Keeping up with the changing external factors in this complicated organizational environment is no easy feat. Decisions made by leaders to address or adapt to these external factors can have unintended adverse effects on health care providers—a trickle-down, or downstream, effect.

In Chapter 3 we discussed the factors related to the individual physician that increase the risk of burnout. In Chapters 4 through 7, we covered the factors within the practice environment that put pressure on physicians and can lead to burnout. In this chapter, we will examine the factors outside the health care workplace that put pressure on organizations and raise the stress level within the practice environment, increasing the risk of burnout. These external factors—and leaders' responses to them—significantly impact the health care workplace.

For simplicity we've divided the external drivers into three categories: flaws in the health system infrastructure, social and demographic changes, and changes related to health reform.

## FLAWS IN THE HEALTH SYSTEM INFRASTRUCTURE

Why are health care workplaces so poorly designed that they create toxic environments that foster burnout? A lot has to do with the way the health care delivery system is structured. The US health care system was not designed with intention; instead it formed incrementally over time. As new initiatives or regulations are implemented, the response of the parties affected—hospitals, health systems, and physician groups—is layered onto the existing system. No overarching entity enacted a thoughtful redesign that took into account all existing requirements and the associated downstream consequences. The result is that health care organizations have not been designed with the intention to function effectively in the current environment. (There are a few exceptions, which we will discuss in Chapter 10.) As Jack Billi told us, "The health care system and its individual processes were not designed, they just evolved. For that reason, there are countless opportunities for improvement to eliminate error, delays, and rework."

Leaders of health care organizations have reacted to each new change in the external environment as an isolated event, resulting in dysfunctional workflows. The broken processes are evident at the microsystem level of a single office visit for a limited problem and at the macrosystem level of complex interventional care for a chronic disease provided over time and in multiple settings. With the pressure to increase throughput and productivity constantly growing, clinical teams are rarely able to step back and evaluate their workflow to understand when a fix for one problem has had unintended consequences.

Along with the lack of a solidly built infrastructure, the health care system is not reliable. To put this lack of reliability into perspective, consider two other complex, high-stakes professions: aviation and nuclear energy. By adopting standard practices and employing strategies to identify and mitigate mistakes, these industries now achieve error rates that are exponentially lower than those currently achieved in health care. (Nolan 2000; Nolan 2004) In short, the health care system was not built to catch errors before they harm a patient or to prevent such errors reliably. As Atul Gawande wrote in a 2011 *New Yorker* article, "It's like no one's in charge—because no one is…We train, hire, and pay doctors to be cowboys. But it's pit crews people need." (Gawande 2011)

Another persistent flaw in the health care system is the tendency to impose changes on workers rather than engaging them in problem-solving and the design of solutions. This oversight reflects a lack of trust in the capabilities of frontline workers. While not universal, Paul's experience suggests that many health care systems are not yet ready to engage the front lines of the health care workforce in problem-solving and redesign.

Finally, an important external factor that relates to the health care system as a whole is the malpractice climate in the United States. The risk of a malpractice suit remains a concern for many physicians. The risk varies by specialty, geographic location, and employer. It is significant enough in some specialties, such as neurosurgery and obstetrics/gynecology, to result in physician shortages in some regions, as physicians have chosen to stop practicing high-risk specialties or leave high-risk locations. The risk of a lawsuit has not changed much in the past 20 years, but the devastating personal impact can lead to burnout, even if the case is ultimately decided in the physician's favor. Research has shown that physicians with a recent malpractice claim are more likely to experience burnout, depression, and thoughts of suicide. (Balsh 2010)

## SOCIAL AND DEMOGRAPHIC CHANGES

Our society is dynamic. Social and demographic shifts affect the demand for health care services. The most important changes in recent years are increasing longevity, the aging of the baby boomer generation, the growing cultural and linguistic diversity of the population with increasing recognition of the need for cultural sensitivity, and the increasing prevalence of chronic diseases such as diabetes, obesity, cardiovascular disease, and HIV-AIDS.

Our society is rapidly aging. Baby boomers are becoming seniors at a rate of 10,000 per day. (Pew 2010) Older people present to physicians' offices with more complex clinical situations. Patients now have more diagnoses, are taking more medications (including over-the-counter medicines that previously required prescriptions and an ever-expanding selection of alternative medications), and have more complex histories. They have often survived cancer, heart attacks, or various surgeries.

Our society is also more diverse. More patients who are not native English speakers present for care than in the past, and health care providers are now required to offer translation services. This requirement reduces the risk of errors yet adds time to the visit as the history and treatment plans must be translated, either by an in-person translator or over a speaker phone using a translation service. In addition, cultural differences in seeking care, describing symptoms, and permitting examinations often result in additional work for care providers or uncertainty about diagnoses and treatment plans.

## CHANGES IN PATIENT EXPECTATIONS

Patient expectations about care have changed. Thanks to the Internet, patients have greater access to health information, whether accurate or not. Patient advocacy groups have increased the engagement and empowerment of many patients. Richard Davies deBronkart, Jr., widely known on the Internet as e-Patient Dave, exemplifies the expansion of patient activism. Through social media, he has advocated for transformation of the health care system to include the active participation of patients in their health and health care and to include patients' rights regarding personal health data. (deBronkart 2016)

In addition, the marketing efforts of health care systems have influenced patient expectations. As systems compete to attract new patients, they develop and market "centers of excellence" in various clinical competencies such as cardiovascular or cancer care. Marketing sets an expectation that the care delivered in these centers is world-class, but often the operations are not designed to deliver on that promise. When a patient has a care experience that is inconsistent with what the marketing promise led him or her to expect, it can result in distrust of the system and of the provider working in the system, which makes the physician's effort to create a healing relationship that much more challenging.

Tiffany Christensen, double-lung-transplant patient, patient advocate, and performance improvement specialist at the North Carolina Quality Center, recognizes that challenge. She told us, "It's not that patients' expectations are unrealistic to want, but that they are unrealistic based on what care providers can deliver in the current system. In my experience, care providers often believe that building rapport and collaborating with patients will take a lot more time, which is not the case. Often, what's needed are concrete skills, like motivational interviewing." Christensen believes that the adversarial relationship that can develop when patients' expectations aren't met can contribute to physician burnout.

## EXPANDED ACCESS TO CARE

Fewer patients today are concerned about continuity of care with their primary care physician than in the past. (Bryant 2016) As physicians are working shifts and protecting their personal time, patients are more willing to see doctors, nurse practitioners, or physician assistants who are available when it is convenient rather than wait to see their primary care physician. Access during non-traditional hours has expanded as a result. In some cases, appointment slots between 6:00 a.m. and 8:00 a.m. fill faster than traditional hours or appointments after 5:00 p.m. Many offices are now open on Saturdays, and some specialists are offering scheduled appointments on Sundays. These changes in scheduling and available hours affect patients, but they also affect physicians and other care providers, lengthening the work day and adding complexity to scheduling.

## WORKFORCE SHORTAGES

Shortages in nursing staff have been an issue for many years. In 2008, the American Association of Colleges of Nursing estimated a vacancy rate of about 8 percent—a deficit of about 135,000 registered nurses. (AACN 2014) The shortage is expected to grow substantially, as baby boomer nurses retire, to 260,000 registered nurses by 2025. (Buerhaus 2009) In Paul's experience coaching in a number of health care systems around the country, he has observed vacancy rates for nursing positions of up to 25 percent.

The supply of physicians in the United States has fluctuated over recent decades. (IOM 2004) However, when the overall number of physicians has been adequate, the geographic distribution has not matched the need, especially in rural areas. (IOM 2004) Looking ahead, several entities have predicted that physician shortages are likely, despite the fact that the applicant pool for residency positions increased by 33 percent between 2002 and 2012. (IOM 2004) The American Association of Medical Colleges has estimated a deficit of up to 90,000 physicians by 2025. (AAMC 2015) Shortages are predicted to be especially severe in primary care fields. The Health Resources and Services Administration has projected a shortfall of 20,400 primary care physicians in 2020.

(HRSA 2013) Ideally, more medical students would choose primary care, and family medicine residency programs would expand accordingly. However, many factors discourage students from choosing primary care specialties, including long hours and lower compensation than in other specialties. Because it takes up to a decade to train physicians, immediate correction is required if the United States is to avert these shortages. (AAMC 2015)

## GENERATIONAL DIFFERENCES IN PRIORITIES

On the whole, physicians of the millennial generation are more likely to prioritize work-life balance. The choice to limit work hours to achieve balance benefits these physicians personally and may reduce the risk of burnout. As baby boomer physicians retire, however, work hours reduction by millennials will compound physician shortages: it takes about 1.5 millennial physicians to replace a baby boomer who worked 60 to 80 hours a week. (Young 2016)

## CHANGES RELATED TO HEALTH REFORM

The cost efficiency, safety, and quality of the health care system all have a huge impact on our lives. The current status of the US system leaves much to be desired.

- Health care in the United States is expensive. It consumes 17.1 percent of the GDP, twice the amount of any other developed country. (World Bank 2016) Health care also consumes a significant portion of our personal income and exacts a substantial financial burden on many families. (Cohen 2014)
- Health care in the United States is not safe enough. In 1999 the Institute of Medicine estimated that there were 98,000 deaths annually due to medical error annually. (IOM 1999) More recent estimates indicate that this figure may have underestimated the true number of deaths due to medical errors. (James 2013) A recent study in the *British Medical Journal* assessed the contribution of medical error to deaths in the United States, including

causes that are not captured in death certificate information. The analysis suggests that medical error is the third-leading cause of death in the United States. (Makary 2016)

- Health care in the United States fails to achieve great patient outcomes. (Berwick, 2008; McCarthy 2011) Our well-being depends on the quality, safety, and coordination of the services we receive. In addition, the personal interactions we have with doctors and other care providers have a significant effect on our ability to make lifestyle changes to maintain health and prevent disease.
- Health care in the United States is time-consuming. Time spent accessing care diverts time from other activities. In 2010, people in the United States spent 1.1 billion hours seeking health care for themselves or for loved ones. (Ray 2015) That time is estimated to have cost the United States economy $52 billion in lost wages.

Health care experts have called for widespread improvement. Many focus on the goal of achieving the Triple Aim: "improving the experience of care, improving the health of populations, and reducing per capita costs of health care." (Berwick 2008) The overarching goal of health reform is to improve these elements of the health care system. State and local authorities and the federal government have been focused on reducing the cost of care. Legislators have imposed a litany of cost-related regulations on health care payers and providers to try to slow the escalation of costs and increase the value of the care provided for the dollars spent. In addition, large employers, whose bottom line is significantly affected by health care costs, have become more proactive in establishing restrictions regarding how provider organizations are paid, which influences where patients receive care (for example, referral to a center of excellence across the country) and other aspects of care delivery.

The aspirational goals of health reform, namely, improvements in cost, quality, and safety, are clearly needed. However, redesign of such a large, complex system, which cannot be taken "off-line" for repairs, is very challenging. To fix what's broken while continuing to provide care is like trying to change the tires on a bus while continuing to drive it down the road. In addition, any change can induce stress, and the transition period between the old and the new is especially problematic. Health reform initiatives have spawned secondary effects that impact physicians' career paths and their daily experiences. Two areas in which health reform has induced change for physicians are finance and new regulatory requirements.

## CHANGES RELATED TO FINANCE

The most obvious changes of health reform are those related to finance. These changes are driven by federal legislation, specifically the ACA and MACRA; pressure from governmental and private payers to shift to payment based on value; and a spate of mergers, acquisitions, and new providers.

The shift from volume to value is evident in several initiatives: high-deductible health plans, which put the patient more at risk for the first dollar of the cost of care; accountable care organizations and capitation agreements, which pay for services for a determined population; bundled payment programs, which reimburse for a determined episode of care; and state-specific insurance exchanges, which facilitate the purchase of health insurance in accordance with the ACA.

**ACA.** The Patient Protection and Affordable Care Act of 2010 (ACA) ushered in significant changes for health care providers. The ACA requires that most US citizens and legal residents have health insurance, includes individual and employer mandates regarding coverage with potential premium subsidies, and creates state-based mechanisms to provide coverage, primarily through insurance exchanges and expansion of Medicaid. It establishes regulations regarding baseline requirements for benefits offered by insurance plans and consumer protections. Importantly, the ACA also supports new approaches to delivering and financing care—including bundled payments for episodes of care, improving chronic disease care, and expanding preventive services—and provides funding for innovation projects to test new modes of health care delivery.

The ACA has expanded access for patients, especially to primary care services, but has adversely affected the physician-patient relationship in a variety of ways. As hospital payments have become dependent on patient satisfaction scores, hospitals have begun to pressure physicians to ensure that every patient is happy with his or her encounter. At times this emphasis results in a conflict for the physician—for example, when deciding how to meet a patient's request for tests or treatments that are not indicated for the diagnosis. In addition, many new insurance options include a high deductible, putting the patient at direct financial risk for the cost of care. Patients are increasingly balking at the cost of recommended care and asking their physicians to offer less-expensive alternatives. These changes increase the stress and clerical tasks involved with patient care.

**MACRA.** The Medicare Access and CHIP Reauthorization Act (MACRA) of 2015 is the largest reform of payment policy since the initiation of the resource-based relative value scale (RBRVS) system for the Medicare fee schedule in 1989. MACRA repeals the use of the sustainable growth rate (SGR) methodology for determining updates to the Medicare physician fee schedule. It establishes the Merit-based Incentive Payment System (MIPS), which consolidates existing Medicare quality programs and provides for adjustments in payment to providers based on quality performance, starting at 4 percent in 2019 and increasing to 9 percent by 2022. MACRA also establishes a pathway for physicians to participate in an alternative payment model (APM), including accountable care organizations (ACOs) and bundled payment programs. MACRA has provided a quality performance program for the largest health care payer in the United States and has broadened the scope of value-based payment programs.

Although moving from volume-based to value-based reimbursement will improve the alignment of incentives in the health care system, the associated regulations require that physicians understand the intricacies of the reimbursement programs to ensure they are able to meet the requirements and thus avoid revenue loss. Understanding and complying with the regulations represents a significant increase in administrative tasks for many physician practices, whether in solo offices or large groups.

**Value-based payment.** The desire of governmental and private payers to curtail escalating costs ushered in a new approach to providing and reimbursing for care: one that pays based on the value of care provided rather than on the number of procedures, tests, and exams performed. With the shift to value-based payment, many hospitals are moving from fee-for-service (FFS), in which hospitals benefit from offering more expensive, high-tech services such as advanced imaging modalities and robotics surgery, to payment based on population health management, in which they benefit from caring for more patients. The shift in focus requires that hospitals expand their reach to more communities and to more sub-populations within these communities.

The shift away from FFS is new territory and has led to confusion and uncertainty about the risk and about the optimal timing for moving away from traditional payment models. Adding to the challenge is the fact that the term *value* is defined differently based on one's vantage point. Value from a population-health standpoint is derived from reducing the cost of care for defined populations of patients and improving health outcomes. Value from an individual patient's standpoint is derived from paying the least amount possible for the most convenient service with the highest quality, essentially making health care a retail experience. Both of these perspectives are actively at play in the current environment. To succeed, health care providers must act according to two different playbooks: one that considers the overall health and costs of their panel of patients and one that prioritizes high-quality, safe, compassionate care for the patient sitting in their office or lying on their exam table.

According to Stephen M. Shortell, PhD, MPH, MBA, dean emeritus and professor at the School of Public Health and Haas School of Business at the University of California, Berkeley, health care organizations are failing to support physicians in making the relevant shifts in practice to adapt to the changes related to health reform. "In the midst of so many changes in how to deliver care, providers are not getting enough help from organizations to make the changes, putting them at risk for burnout."

Sue Cejka at Grant Cooper Healthcare described to us the dilemma for physicians and leaders of provider organizations. "A lot of my clients are in trouble. They have one foot in the fee-for-service world and one foot in population health. They will lose money until they are all on one side or the other. Take, for example, a 58-year-old physician who knows the patient well and has the clinical confidence to order fewer tests and procedures. Having an experienced physician is better for the patient, but is it better for the organization? It depends. In fee-for-service, it reduces revenues. In capitation, it saves money."

Municipalities are beginning to recognize the importance of controlling health care costs. Whereas local governments traditionally attract new businesses by highlighting quality-of-life amenities and offering tax breaks, now employers are evaluating workforce health care costs as a significant corporate expense and are weighing these costs as a factor in deciding where to locate their offices and factories. Recognizing the impact of health care costs, municipalities and employers are redesigning health benefits accordingly, which has increased the pressure on hospitals and health systems to reduce costs.

Research has demonstrated that the shift from volume to value has decreased the rate of escalation of health care spending. A 2015 study found that in the first year of Maryland's experiment in setting all-payer rates for hospital services, per capita hospital costs decreased by 1.08 percent in Maryland, while nationally these costs increased by 1.07 percent, translating into a cost savings of $116 million. (Patel 2015)

**Mergers, acquisitions, and new providers.** Legislative and regulatory changes related to health reform have accelerated the trend toward mergers and acquisitions of health care entities that was previously well underway.

These include:

- Mergers of large systems with each other
- Mergers of hospitals into health systems
- Mergers of medical groups into hospital systems
- Mergers of medical groups with each other
- Mergers of small or solo practices into larger groups
- Acquisition of smaller hospitals, medical groups, and small or solo practices by larger entities

These changes in ownership have substantially increased the number of physicians who work as employees of larger entities rather than as sole proprietors of small businesses. As we discussed in Chapters 4 and 5, these changes directly affect the key drivers of burnout, especially the degree of control over work.

Another significant shift in the health care market is the entrance of new providers. For example, Walgreens, CVS, and Target have developed models to deliver short-term care for acute problems and complex chronic diseases through retail clinics in their stores.

Two of the most obvious effects of health reform on physicians, increased cost consciousness and productivity pressure, demand a different way of practicing medicine—one that most physicians were not anticipating when they entered medical school and have not been trained to adopt. In addition, when leaders focus primarily on these aspects of organizational performance while minimizing the importance of other metrics on a balanced dashboard, the resulting operational decisions significantly affect physicians. Dike Drummond, the physician coach and consultant, told us, "When I ask the doctors in a 500-physician hospital how many of the hospital's new initiatives in the past year related to improving their practice experience, the answer is, 'None.' They are all driven by external mandates." Substantiating this focus on productivity metrics is a recent study of executive-level health care leaders in the United States and Canada. When asked whether they include burnout and well-being of employees and physicians in their process improvement metrics, only 17 percent of respondents replied affirmatively. (Boehm 2015)

## NEW REGULATORY REQUIREMENTS

In addition to new regulations related to the ACA and MACRA, health care organizations and care providers are dealing with a variety of new regulatory requirements. Those with the greatest impact on physicians include ICD-10, Meaningful Use, and additional professional certification requirements.

**Diagnostic coding with ICD-10.** The International Classification of Diseases (ICD), a classification system developed by the World Health Organization, has evolved over time, reflecting the growth in medical knowledge. The ICD represents the standard for identifying ailments and injuries and provides a numerical code for every diagnosis. Although most of the developed world has been using ICD-10 codes for a number of years, US physicians had been using the previous version until the fall of 2015. ICD-10 introduced several significant changes, such as:

- Increasing the maximum number of digits in each code from 5 to 7
- Increasing the number of codes from 14,000 to 69,000
- Adding laterality where applicable (for example, injury to the right side vs. left side)
- Adding severity parameters
- Adding combination codes to designate complexity

These changes allow actuaries and health policy workers to better identify, understand, and analyze patterns of illness and injury. Many physicians question whether the benefits to population health are worth the additional burden that generating the codes places on physicians—especially when they are already feeling overworked. These physicians find the extra work particularly irritating because it has little to do with the actual care of patients. As one hospitalist who left practice because of burnout explained to us, "Spending so much time looking for billable items to code didn't seem to be what I should be doing. It was not related to how happy or well you make the patient feel. There was a huge disconnect between what I wanted to be doing and what I was actually doing."

**Meaningful Use incentive program.** From the time of their development in the early 1990s, the use of EHRs grew slowly until the HITECH Act of 2009. The Act implemented, through the Meaningful Use initiative, incentives to providers for EHR adoption starting in 2011, with the threat of penalties for failure to adopt EHRs by 2015. The three-stage incentive program catalyzed a rapid expansion of the computerization of medical records, including electronic progress notes and orders. As a federal program, Meaningful Use is clearly an external factor. Note that we covered the EHR in great depth in the last chapter because of its profound effect on the daily practice and workplace of physicians.

**Additional professional certification requirements.** Most medical groups, hospitals, and insurance companies require that physicians maintain certification in their specialty. Such certification requires graduation from medical school, completion of residency training, and successfully passing a specialty board exam, which may include written and oral case presentations. The American Board of Medical Specialties (ABIM) oversees the certification process, by which national specialty organizations grant "board certification."

The ABIM designed the certification process to ensure a minimum standard of knowledge for practicing physicians. In the last few decades, though, most specialty boards have begun requiring ongoing certification with a periodic exam every seven to ten years. Some specialties have added further requirements, including documentation of quality improvement activity in the physician's practice or more frequent testing on specific areas of focus within a specialty. The required activities and the associated documentation have become increasingly complex; as a result, some specialty boards are now considering reducing the additional requirements.

The combination of coding, computer, and certification requirements has translated into a substantial increase in the amount of time physicians spend on non-clinical tasks. According to Wayne Sotile at the Center for Physician Resilience, these tasks are a key contributor to burnout among physicians. "I see physicians who are overwhelmed with a landslide of documentation demands. Most spend two to three hours a day on documentation alone." Karen Weiner at the Oregon Medical Group concurs. "The effects of mandates related to health reform are enormous. I see very low morale in physicians, especially those in adult primary care."

∬∬

Physician burnout is a predictable response to working in stressful, broken systems and unsupportive work environments, created in part due to the external drivers described in this chapter. Although real prevention requires fixing the underlying root problems and creating healthy workplaces, interventions aimed at individual physicians, such as coaching, mindfulness, and stress reduction, can mitigate stressors. In Part 3, we'll begin our discussion of solutions by focusing on available individually focused interventions.

## REFERENCES

American Association of Colleges of Nursing. Nursing shortage. 2014. Available at: http://www.aacn.nche.edu/media-relations/fact-sheets/nursing-shortage. Accessed June 5, 2016.

American Association of Medical Colleges. The complexities of physician supply and demand: projections from 2013 to 2025. 2015. Available at: https://www.aamc.org/download/426242/data/ihsreportdownload.pdf?cm_mmc=AAMC-_-ScientificAffairs-_-PDF-_-ihsreport. Accessed June 5, 2016.

Balsh CM, Oreskovich MR, Dyrbye LN, et al. Personal consequences of malpractice lawsuits on American surgeons. *J Am Coll Surg.* 2011;213:657–667.

Berwick DM, Nolan TW, Whittington J. The Triple Aim: care, health, and cost. *Health Aff.* 2008;27(3):759–769.

Boehm L, Petty K. Humanizing efficiency in health care. 2015. Vocera Experience Innovation Network. Available at: http://solutions.vocera.com/rs/742-LCM-112/images/2015_11%20Humanizing%20Efficiency%20electronic%20final.pdf. Accessed June 6, 2016.

Bryant M. Here come the millennials: what providers need to know. [Internet]. 2016. Available at: http://www.healthcaredive.com/news/here-come-the-millennials-what-providers-need-to-know/419037/. Accessed July 8, 2016.

Buerhaus PI, Auerbach DI, Staiger DO. The recent surge in nurse employment: causes and implications. *Health Aff.* 2009;28(4):w657–w668.

Cohen RA, Kirzinger WK. Financial burden of medical care: A family perspective. NCHS data brief, no 142. Hyattsville, MD: National Center for Health Statistics. 2014.

E-Patient Dave: A voice of patient empowerment: about. 2016. Available at: http://www.epatientdave.com/about-dave. Accessed June 5, 2016.

Gawande A. Cowboys and pit crews. 2011. *New Yorker.* Available at: http://www.newyorker.com/news/news-desk/cowboys-and-pit-crews. Accessed June 5, 2016.

Health Resources and Services Administration, National Center for Health Workforce Analysis. Projecting the supply and demand for primary care practitioners through 2020. 2013. Available at: http://

bhpr.hrsa.gov/healthworkforce/supplydemand/usworkforce/primarycare/. Accessed June 5, 2016.

Institute of Medicine. *Graduate Medical Education that Meets the Nation's Health Needs.* Washington, DC: The National Academies Press. 2014.

Institute of Medicine. *To Err Is Human: Building a Safer Health Care System.* Washington, DC: National Academies Press. 1999.

James JT. A new, evidence-based estimate of patient harms associated with hospital care. *J Patient Saf.* 2013;9(3):122–128.

Makary MA, Daniel M. Medical error—the third leading cause of death in the US. *BMJ.* 2016;353:i2139. Available at: http://www.bmj.com/content/353/bmj.i2139. Accessed July 8, 2016.

McCarthy D, How SKH, Fryer AK, Radley D, Schoen C. *The Commonwealth Fund Commission on a High Performance Health System, Why Not the Best? Results from the National Scorecard on US Health System Performance, 2011.* New York: The Commonwealth Fund. 2011.

Nolan T. System changes to improve patient safety. *BMJ.* 2000;320:771–773.

Nolan T, Resar R, Haraden C, Griffom FA. Improving the reliability of health care. Institute for Healthcare Improvement. 2004. Available at: http://www.ihi.org/education/IHIOpenSchool/Courses/Documents/CourseraDocuments/08_ReliabilityWhitePaper2004revJune06.pdf. Accessed June 5, 2016.

Patel A, Rajkumar R, Colmers JM, Kinzer D, Conway PH, Sharfstein JM. Maryland's global hospital budgets—preliminary results from an all-payer model. *N Engl J Med.* 2015;373:1899–1901.

Pew Research. Baby boomers retire. 2010. Available at: http://www.pewresearch.org/daily-number/baby-boomers-retire. Accessed June 5, 2016.

Ray KN, Chari AV, Engberg J, Bertolet M, Mehrotra A. Opportunity costs of ambulatory medical care in the United States. *Am J Manag Care.* 2015;21(8):567–574.

Sinsky C. Redesigning the practice model for general internal medicine: a proposal for coordinated care. *J Gen Intern Med.* 2007;22:400–409.

The World Bank. Health expenditure, total (% of GDP): 2011–2015. 2016. Available at: http://data.worldbank.org/indicator/SH.XPD.TOTL.ZS. Accessed June 5, 2016.

Young J. Millennial providers and work-life balance: are they on to something? CEP America. 2016. Available at: http://www.cepamerica. com/news-resources/perspectives-on-the-acute-care-continuum/ march-2016/millennial-providers-work-life-balance. Accessed June 5, 2016.

# PART 3
## PREVENTING PHYSICIAN BURNOUT

We firmly believe that preventing burnout requires attention to the three levels at which drivers exist, as we described in Part 2: the individual physician, the workplace, and the environment external to the workplace. All three levels must be addressed to create optimal patient-physician interactions and build sustainable careers for physicians.

Many health care organizations and wellness coaches have emphasized prevention strategies aimed at the individual level—strategies that focus primarily on building the resilience of the physician to stress. The emphasis on these programs may reflect the erroneous belief that burnout is caused by individual susceptibility. Alternatively, it may reflect the fact that it is easier to launch a wellness program than it is to identify and address the underlying systems problems. Leading change in patient care workflows, management systems, and organizational culture is challenging work that requires the ability to guide the technical and the emotional aspects of change. The focus on wellness programs may also reflect a sincere desire on the part of health care leaders to provide hope and solace to physicians in the short term, while searching for more definitive solutions.

According to Christina Maslach, formerly at the University of California, Berkeley, the focus on wellness programs to address burnout is concerning. "Organizations are creating programs to help people cope, but it begs the question: How about changing something about what they are coping with? What's going wrong with the world of work? I worry that wellness programs are being framed as solutions to burnout, when actually there is a lot more going on in the workplace. So why not tweak the work environment? Let's try some things that might lessen the burden on people, so we don't have to spend so much time on trying to fix, cure, and treat them afterwards" (personal communication, February 1, 2016).

Although individual strategies are important to ensure that the physician is at his or her best when providing patient care, in the long run, these strategies cannot prevent the effects of continuous exposure to chaotic, inefficient, stressful work environments. In addition, leaders who implement wellness programs based on individual strategies without addressing the deep concerns of physicians run the risk of alienating care providers who see the wellness initiative as a token effort and a failure of administration to fix their real concerns.

The evidence base regarding the prevalence of and risk factors for burnout is somewhat established, but the data about effective interventions for burnout are much less robust. A recent analysis of published studies found few randomized, controlled trials, a range of modestly effective interventions, and no clear difference in benefits among the various interventions studied. (West 2016) Given the lack of definitive evidence, we highlight initiatives currently under way and offer suggestions based on the known causes of burnout.

Addressing burnout includes treatment for acute symptoms and strategies for prevention. In the next chapter, we'll describe some of the individual strategies for treating acute burnout and building resiliency to help prevent burnout. Then, in subsequent chapters, we'll focus on strategies to fix the root causes of burnout in the workplace. We devote an entire chapter to leadership, because research and our experience have shown that effective leadership is essential for creating a workplace and organizational culture in which health care providers can thrive.

We will conclude, in our final chapter, with recommendations for action steps for physicians and for leaders.

We do not propose in this book any actions to address the external drivers. Policy and advocacy work is critical for making long-term improvements, but that is beyond the scope of our work and expertise. We do believe that while we await improvements in external drivers, much can be done today to alleviate the problems that are making clinical careers unsustainable for too many physicians.

## REFERENCE

West CP, Dyrbye LN, Erwin PJ, Shanafelt TD. Interventions to prevent and reduce physician burnout: a systematic review and meta-analysis. *Lancet.* 2016;388:2272–2281.

# CHAPTER 9

## INDIVIDUAL APPROACHES AND WELLNESS PROGRAMS

*Self-care is not selfish. In coaching, I try to change
the physician's mind set to allow for self-care.*
—STARLA FITCH, MD, OCULOPLASTIC SURGEON,
PHYSICIAN COACH, AND AUTHOR

*I had a near-burnout experience in training. But I
was fortunate. I sought counseling and developed
an effective coping mechanism: running. When I felt
exhausted or overwhelmed, I would leave the hospital,
go for a run, and come back later to finish my notes.*
—GENE LINDSEY, MD, FORMER PRESIDENT
AND CEO OF ATRIUS HEALTH

I n this chapter we'll address approaches for preventing burnout that
are focused on individual physicians. First, however, we want to discuss treatment for physicians with acute burnout. Given the suffering
caused by untreated burnout and the increased risk of suicide among
physicians, identifying physicians with acute burnout and assisting them
in promptly accessing needed care is an absolute necessity.

## TREATMENT FOR ACUTE BURNOUT

Physicians who are experiencing severe, acute burnout need immediate help. They and their patients are at risk for the many negative

consequences described in Chapter 2. This section provides an overview of some of the interventions available for physicians with acute burnout. These interventions include time away from work, professional assistance programs, counseling, coaching, and suicide prevention strategies.

## Time away from work

For a physician suffering from the acute effects of burnout, which can include cognitive problems, as we described in Chapter 2, a period of time away from work may be necessary for recuperation. As UK psychotherapist Zoë Krupka, PhD, said in an online post in 2015, "No amount of multivitamins, yoga, meditation, sweaty exercise, superfoods, or extreme time management, as brilliant as all these things can be, is going to save us from the effects of too much work." (Krupka 2015)

Physician-author Tom Murphy, MD, found that a break from working was essential for healing from the effects of burnout. After about two years, Murphy returned to work. About his return, he said, "[I am] back into practice and it's joyful rather than what medicine had become for me." (Murphy 2015)

Time off can be structured in different ways, depending on the physician's personal circumstances and the benefits policy of the organization for which he or she works. As such, the time may be a paid or unpaid leave of absence, a paid sabbatical, vacation time, or medical leave. Unfortunately, even when a physician has come forward for help, his or her organization may not recognize the urgency of the need and respond accordingly.

One coach that Diane interviewed shared a disturbing story about a client. The physician, who was in his early 60s, was experiencing severe burnout, with cognitive effects that were affecting his ability to make decisions. The physician's psychiatrist and personal physician recommended a three-month leave. He approached the administration of the hospital, revealed the situation, and requested an unpaid leave. His request was rejected. Administration cited the ongoing demand for physicians, saying, "We need you to be seeing patients."

## Professional assistance

Physicians with acute burnout may need professional assistance. Comorbid conditions, such as substance abuse, anxiety, and depression, often accompany burnout and require specific treatment. Sources of help include individual, family, and couples' counselors, substance abuse professionals, physician support services through the local or state medical society, and employee assistance programs.

Most states in the country maintain a physician health program (PHP), although the services offered and the confidentiality policies vary. In many cases, information about physicians who enter PHPs voluntarily remains confidential. However, state licensure and credentialing applications generally require disclosure of any condition that might impair practice, including substance abuse and mental health conditions. PHPs can provide evaluations, appropriate referrals for treatment, and monitoring for substance use. Many physicians remain leery of voluntarily entering PHPs due to fear of the potential impact on their career. (For more information, see the Federation of State Physician Health Programs at www.fsphp.org.)

## Counseling

Professional counseling with a social worker, psychologist, or psychiatrist is critical for physicians with a co-existing mental health condition and can be very helpful for other physicians as well. Some organizations have developed physician-specific assistance programs to address the particular counseling needs of physicians.

More than a decade ago, Adventist Health System, a 46-hospital health system headquartered in central Florida, began offering professional counseling with an in-house psychologist to physicians and their family members. In the 12 years since its inception, the program has provided more than 10,000 visits to more than 750 physicians and 250 family members. According to Ted Hamilton of Adventist Health System the program has been well-received, highly used, and effective. As he said, "I can't tell what [the program has] done for marriages, careers, and having kinder, healthier doctors walking the halls, but I am absolutely convinced it's immense."

Wayne Sotile of the Center for Physician Resilience has provided counseling to physicians and their families for more than 30 years. He told us that he brings his training in family systems therapy to bear when working with physicians: "Individual physicians won't sustain their improvement in counseling without changes in the family system. We bring the physician's spouse in to sessions and work with the American Medical Association Alliance to impact medical families. You cannot curb burnout without creating a resilient physician and a resilient family system."

Sotile also sees the value of *targeted* coaching for physicians with burnout and their families. "After 30-plus years of practice, I am convinced that the vast majority of physicians do not require formal mental health intervention to curb burnout. They require coaching to broaden and deepen their abilities to cope with change, navigate work and family dynamics, and appropriately care for themselves. And they need this training to be targeted and practical." The Center provides one- to four-day intensives in which physicians (with or without their spouses) receive individualized coaching. "We work with one physician or one medical family at a time, intensively, and follow-up remotely."

Finally, Sotile emphasizes the importance of addressing the work environment. "Neither physicians nor medical families will remain resilient if the physician's workplace is toxic. Our career paths epitomize this point. We've moved over the decades from working with individual physicians, to working with medical families, to working with medical organizations—trying to get everyone on the same page."

Counseling can help physicians with acute burnout to identify and begin to address current stressors as well as substance abuse and co-morbid mental health conditions.

## Coaching

An executive or personal coach can help a physician with burnout identify precipitating factors and make decisions that support his or her recovery. Some coaches specialize in helping physicians; many of these professionals are physicians who left practice themselves or continue to practice on a reduced schedule. Coaching can offer an individualized approach with support, mentorship, and the ability to learn from the experience of others. Starla Fitch, MD, oculoplastic surgeon, physician coach, and author of *Remedy for Burnout: 7 Prescriptions Doctors Use to Find Meaning in Medicine*, told us that her focus for identifying solutions is on the individual physician. "I start with the individual and work from the inside out. I ask the physician, 'What changes can you make within the system?'"

A significant part of that change relates to time management and delegation of tasks, according to Fitch. She helps the physician break down the day and identify tasks that he or she can eliminate. She also shares examples from her own life. "I asked my secretary to fill in the rote parts of the form for my oculoplastic procedures. Over the course of a week, it saves me half an hour." With her clients, Fitch emphasizes the need to let go of the "we can do it all" attitude, saying, "It's okay to ask others for help. It's okay to say, 'I can't bake cupcakes for my child's second-grade class,' and ask for help with the baking or bring store-bought treats."

Fitch believes that coaching offers several benefits to physicians with burnout. She explained, "It allows them to be deeply heard, gives them time to think about their world and take a breath, gives them a sounding board to know their requests are not unreasonable, and it gives them mentoring in 'how to do my life.'"

Michelle Mudge-Riley, the career coach, listed similar benefits to coaching. She told us, "Coaching is effective because it is an individualized solution. It offers support and mentorship. Sharing the experience with others enables and empowers physicians to find the causes of their burnout and then find solutions." Among the physicians who work with Mudge-Riley, about one-fifth leave practice entirely. The rest continue to practice, but many choose to reduce their practice hours to make space for other endeavors, such as starting a business (for example, a medical concierge service), doing quality or regulatory work, and writing fiction or writing for medical publications.

## Suicide prevention strategies

As we mentioned in Chapter 2, physicians are at higher risk for suicide than are members of the general population. Physicians and organizational leaders can take steps to reduce the risk of suicide among physicians and other care providers. First, they can become aware of the risk factors for physicians and the symptoms of distress. According to Elizabeth Bromley, MD, PhD, a researcher at the University of California, Los Angeles, and founder of The Ruth Carr Center for Physician Vitality, which was named for a surgeon who died by suicide, physicians at risk for suicide can present at work with uncharacteristic irritability, carelessness, rage, withdrawal, or sadness. (Bromley 2014) Second, physicians and leaders can address their concern with the physician directly. Bromley suggests scheduling a specific time in the near future to talk with the at-risk physician and asking directly about the presence of suicidal thoughts. A helpful resource with additional information is the National Suicide Prevention Lifeline at www.suicidepreventionlifeline. org or at 1-800-273-TALK.

The American Medical Association recently released an online module on how to identify physicians at risk for suicide and facilitate access to appropriate care. The module includes a list of risk factors and warning signs, as well as suggested wording for speaking with physicians at risk. (See www.stepsforward.org for more information.)

## INDIVIDUAL PREVENTION STRATEGIES

Individual strategies are the key to treating acute burnout symptoms. Individual strategies can also help prevent burnout by building resilience to stress. A physician who is sleep deprived, is physically out of shape, and has few outlets outside of work for rejuvenation will be more susceptible to the stressors that burn out physicians. These stressors include frustration with an ineffective workflow, exhaustion from after-hours documentation work, the loss of a sense of purpose from disrupted communication with patients, and the other factors we discussed in Part 2. Building resilience is like sailing in a sea-worthy craft: it won't stop the raging storm, but it will allow the sailor to stay afloat far better than will a boat with a leak.

We'll describe several individual strategies that can help build resilience to burnout. These include self-care, stress-reduction techniques, mindfulness, counseling, coaching, engaging in new challenges, achieving a healthy work-life balance and financial balance, reconnecting with purpose, peer support, and wellness programs. Note that almost none of these strategies have been well studied for prevention of burnout. However, anecdotes, common sense, and studies in other scenarios suggest that these interventions may be helpful. At a minimum, they are unlikely to cause harm—unless they are applied with the expectation that they alone are sufficient to adequately address physician burnout.

## Self-care

For many physicians, self-care doesn't seem to come naturally. Perhaps it's the personality traits of those of us who enter the profession as well as the training culture that teaches us to de-prioritize or ignore our personal human needs.

Although self-care may not be a natural response for many physicians, they can learn ways to alleviate stress and reduce the risk of burnout by taking care of themselves. They can maintain a healthy diet and activity level. They can make time for hobbies, adequate sleep, and spending time with loved ones. They can preserve time for spiritual practice, if that is important to them. They can prioritize taking breaks during the work day, even if just for a few minutes.

In *Physician Burnout: A Guide to Recognition and Recovery,* Tom Murphy, MD, details his experience of recovering from burnout. He emphasizes the importance of replenishing oneself in preventing burnout. As he put it, "If you conceive of your career and life as a bucket full of water, there are many aspects of modern medicine that cause small holes in the bottom of the container. It is imperative that you maintain the level in your personal bucket with 'bucket fillers,' namely, the activities you love, lest you become completely depleted." (Murphy 2015)

As Sir William Osler, the Canadian physician and one of the founding professors at Johns Hopkins Hospital, admonished, "The young doctor should look about early for an avocation, a pastime, that will take him away from patients, pills, and potions…No [person] is really happy or safe without one, and it makes precious little difference what the outside interest may be—botany, beetles, or butterflies; roses, tulips, or irises;

fishing, mountaineering, or antiquities—anything will do so long as he straddles a hobby and rides it hard." (Osler Symposium 2016)

### Stress reduction techniques

Stress reduction techniques, such as meditation and yoga, can also help alleviate the effects of stressors. A first step for physicians is cultivating an awareness of their personal stress symptoms. When they observe these symptoms, they can take steps to reduce their stress level. As Robert Altman of Sutter Gould Medical Foundation said, "Over time, I've learned to be more sensitive to my symptoms of stress and burnout. I'm aware sooner and can take action steps, so the symptoms are of shorter duration and have less impact on patient interactions and family relationships than in the past."

### Mindfulness

Mindfulness practice is one of the few individual approaches to preventing burnout that has been studied systematically. Jon Kabat-Zinn, PhD, founder of the Mindfulness-Based Stress Reduction Clinic at University of Massachusetts Medical School, has defined mindfulness as engaging in a "nonjudgmental attentiveness to physical and mental processes." (Kabat-Zinn, 1994) In short, it is "present moment awareness." A key aspect of mindfulness is the ability of the individual to monitor and regulate his or her reactions to unanticipated situations, a skill that can be very helpful in clinical situations. (Epstein 2014)

A 2009 study evaluated the effects of a mindfulness program on burnout and empathy in primary care physicians. (Krasner 2009) Physicians learned and then practiced mindfulness techniques over the course of one year. Physicians showed significant improvement in mindfulness, burnout, empathy, mood disturbance, and emotional stability—changes that persisted after the year-long initiative. A more recent study evaluated physicians who were provided with protected time to join small groups that facilitated mindfulness and self-reflection. Participants showed reduction in burnout symptoms and improved engagement in work. (West 2014)

## Counseling

Counseling, as discussed previously, can help minimize stressors. In the context of burnout prevention, counseling might address the effect of work stressors on other aspects of the physician's life, such as marriage, parenting, and avocational goals.

## Coaching

Coaching, as discussed previously, can also help minimize stressors. In the context of burnout prevention, the coaching would focus less on an immediate action plan and more on long-term goals, strategies, and plans.

## Searching out new challenges

Some physicians find that searching out and pursuing a new challenge in their professional life can help stave off the symptoms of burnout. Paul found that taking on leadership roles provided a different opportunity for professional satisfaction. Starla Fitch, the physician coach, found that expanding her professional work to include coaching and speaking while slightly reducing her clinical hours allowed her to recover from burnout and find joy in practice again. A geriatrician that we interviewed affirmed that taking on new challenges was essential to the sustainability of his practice: "Re-inventing yourself can help you get out of a rut. I've found that making a big change in your life—like moving to a whole new practice setting—can be re-invigorating. You must have something you're working toward."

## Work-life balance

For many physicians today, "work-life balance" may sound like an oxymoron—a laudable, but impossible, goal. Given the chaotic work environments in which many physicians practice, pessimism about the idea of balance is understandable. However, attaining a healthier balance between the professional and non-professional aspects of life—often possible with small changes—is an important step in improving resilience to burnout.

As Dike Drummond, the physician coach and author, cautioned physicians in an online article, "The patient cannot always come first. That is a recipe for burnout. Life balance for physicians can only happen when you say 'yes' to the most important things in your life outside of your career—before you do anything else. Whenever you are not with patients, work-life balance depends on putting your life first." (Drummond, no date)

Research has shown that control over schedule and work hours are important predictors of work-life balance and a lower risk of burnout. (Keeton 2007) Maximizing physicians' input into scheduling and increasing the efficiency of the workplace are important ways that leadership can foster improved work-life balance and reduced risk of burnout.

Taking vacation time is an important part of achieving a healthy balance and renewing one's energy for work. Leaders, especially physician leaders, can be instrumental in modeling the importance of time away from work. Some organizations have addressed this problem proactively by adding physician FTEs. Creating a float pool of physicians or hiring a locum tenens physician to cover for vacation time (as well as for illness, parental leave, and other life events) is an investment that can pay for itself through retention of physicians and avoidance of burnout-associated costs.

### Financial balance

Physicians often make financial sacrifices in their young adulthood. During medical school, residency, and fellowship they work long hours for little monetary reward. Many enter the workforce with substantial educational debt, no equity in a home, and little, if any, savings for retirement or their children's education. Once they begin achieving a higher income, some may expand their lifestyle accordingly and subsequently become trapped in a stressful practice situation in order to generate a sufficient income to support that lifestyle. To reduce stresses related to financial pressures and the need to produce an abundant income, physicians might consider whether they can make changes to lighten their financial load. Many benefit from financial counseling.

## Sense of meaning

Many physician leaders we spoke with identified the loss of a sense of meaning in practice as a major factor in burnout among their peers. They believed that refocusing attention on their purpose in becoming care providers could help physicians to appreciate the positive reactions they have with patients and to combat the daily stresses of practice.

Ricardo Guerra, Jr, of Walnut Hill Medical Center touched on the importance of meaning in an interview. He said, "When you're caught in an endless cycle of pushing papers, or pixels in the case of EHR, it becomes very frustrating because it takes you away from what you want to be doing. We aim to create a culture that gives people meaning, letting them know, 'What you do is not only important but is essential to our overall goal of making a difference in people's lives.' We try to reconnect physicians and other caregivers with the higher goal of improving people's lives."

A number of organizations have created formal initiatives to restore joy and meaning to practice. The American Medical Association developed the STEPS Forward program, which provides online modules aimed at improving practice efficiency and restoring joy to patient care.

Rachel Naomi Remens, MD, founder of the Institute for the Study of Health and Illness (ISHI), developed curricula that support paying more attention to the meaning of patient care. The course is offered at more than 70 medical schools to provide "exploration of the time-honored values of service, healing relationship, reverence for life, and compassionate care." (Remens 2012) ISHI also provides help for physicians who want to start ongoing, self-led support groups to create a safe environment for discussion of topics related to the practice of medicine. A description of the groups emphasizes the goal of restoring a sense of meaning to practice: "Over time, the dialogue within a supportive community of colleagues can have the positive effect of deepening each person's heart connection to their day-to-day work and to their patients, as well as to their connection to the lineage of medicine and healing." (Remens 2012)

Ted Hamilton of Adventist Health System told us about the success he's observed with the use of self-led support groups. "A general surgeon at our hospital began a 'Remens' group in his home. After they met for a number of months, I asked him if the group had made a difference. He described how it had changed the way physicians interact with each other, 'I never get consults sent only via EHR anymore. Physicians call me or they stop me in the hall. They ask me about my kids now. The group is changing the culture of the hospital.'"

## Peer support

Peer support can be invaluable to physicians under stress. Both physicians and organizational leaders have a role to play in extending the reach and scope of peer support. Physicians can prioritize time for informal conversations with colleagues. Leaders can help create opportunities for these connections—or, at a minimum, avoid actions that will further undercut camaraderie among physicians.

One form of peer support that can be helpful is facilitated meetings that allow care providers to de-brief after difficult cases. In many health care organizations in the United States and the United Kingdom, "Schwartz Rounds" provide such a protected space. The Schwartz Center for Compassionate Healthcare is a non-profit organization that helps health care organizations convene Schwartz Center Rounds,® which are facilitated, confidential, multidisciplinary meetings where caregivers can talk about the complex emotional and social issues they face in patient care. A 2010 study found that a majority of the care providers who attended multiple sessions reported feeling less isolated and alone in their work. (Lown 2010)

Peer support can also help physicians under stress. In 2008, Brigham and Women's Hospital (BWH) in Boston launched the Brigham and Women's Hospital Center for Professionalism and Peer Support (CPPS), further developing the hospital's programs designed to support clinicians facing a variety of workplace stresses—the primary being involvement in a medical error. (Shapiro 2016) The peer support model at BWH began as a group support model, which they still utilize. They found, however, that physicians too often felt uncomfortable displaying vulnerability in a multidisciplinary group setting. In addition, their research showed that after medical errors, physicians would most like to receive support from a colleague, rather than from a mental health practitioner. (Hu 2011) In 2009, the hospital redesigned the program, adding a one-on-one, physician-to-physician peer support program, in which a peer who has been trained by the CPPS reaches out to offer support to clinicians involved in any events that are likely to be stressful. (Shapiro 2016) For example, the peer supporters make outreach calls to all physicians involved in an adverse event within the hospital.

According to Jo Shapiro, MD, a surgeon at the hospital and the founding director of CPPS, the vast majority of clinicians who are contacted accept the outreach support (personal communication, July 12, 2016). As Shapiro describes in an online article about the program, "We have found that discussing personal vulnerability and overcoming feelings of isolation are best accomplished through interaction with a caring, trained colleague. These interactions can be brief. Their significance and impact comes from normalizing what feels like a unique and isolating experience." (Shapiro 2014) The article ends with this poignant aspiration: "My hope is that the physician culture will evolve to a place where we are more naturally supporting each other in informal ways, where we are less entrenched in our current ways of interacting… Connecting our painful experiences with empathic others is, I believe, the first step toward forgiving ourselves for being human."

## Wellness programs

In response to the surge in physician burnout, many health care organizations have created physician wellness programs. These programs generally offer an array of strategies focused on the individual: exercise and fitness classes, educational workshops about burnout and depression, mindfulness training, information about accessing referrals for treatment, peer support groups, and individual coaching and counseling. Wellness programs are indispensable for physicians and trainees with acute burnout symptoms and can help promote resilience in all clinicians.

We strongly support the development of these programs. Some physicians need immediate support to prevent serious consequences, including suicide. Many physicians need such support to recover sufficiently to be able to engage in personal and organizational change. In addition, while administrators are addressing the underlying problems driving burnout, they can demonstrate their commitment to physicians and other staff by prioritizing the development and support of wellness programs, which can often be implemented more quickly than initiatives to address burnout drivers in the workplace.

♫♫♫

Individual strategies have an important role in building the resilience needed to cope effectively with the stresses inherent in medical practice. However, individual strategies, even when offered as part of a comprehensive wellness program, are insufficient for preventing burnout. Burnout is a systems problem. Practice-level changes are necessary to stop continually exposing care providers to work environments that are overwhelmingly stressful and unsustainable in the long term. In the next chapter, we'll begin to look at strategies for addressing the problems in the practice environment that are burning out physicians.

## REFERENCES

Bromley E. Pediatric ground rounds: physician burnout. [Presentation]. 2014. Available at: http://www.uctv.tv/shows/28597. Accessed June 10, 2016.

Drummond D. Work life balance for doctors: three steps to saying no with grace and power. [Internet]. Available at: https://www.thehappymd.com/blog/bid/290781/Work-Life-Balance-for-Doctors-Three-Steps-to-Saying-NO-with-Grace-and-Power. Accessed June 9, 2016.

Epstein RM. What will it take for physicians to practice mindfully? Promoting quality of care, quality of caring, resilience, and well-being. In: Ie A, Ngnoumen CT, Langer EJ, eds. *The Wiley Blackwell Handbook of Mindfulness, 1st ed.* Hoboken, NJ: John Wiley & Sons. 2014.

Hu YY, Fix ML, Hevelone ND, et al. Physicians' needs in coping with emotional stressors: the case for peer support. *Arch Surg.* 2011;147(3):212–217.

Kabat-Zinn J. *Wherever You Go, There You Are: Mindfulness Meditation in Everyday Life.* New York: Hyperion. 1994.

Keeton K, Fenner DE, Johnson TRB, Hayward RA. Predictors of physician career satisfaction, work life balance, and burnout. *Obstet Gynecol.* 2007;109(4):949–955.

Krasner MS, Epstein RM, Beckman H, et al. Association of an educational program in mindful communication with burnout, empathy, and attitudes among primary care physicians. *JAMA.* 2009;302(12):1284–1293.

Krupka Z. No it's not you. Why wellness is not the answer to overwork. [Internet]. 2015. Available at: http://theconversation.com/no-its-not-you-why-wellness-isnt-the-answer-to-overwork-42124. Accessed June 7, 2016.

Lown BA, Manning CF. The Schwartz Center Rounds: evaluation of an interdisciplinary approach to enhancing patient-centered communication, teamwork, and provider support. *Acad Med.* 2010;85(6):1073–81.

Murphy T. *Physician Burnout: A Guide to Recognition and Recovery.* Aloha Publishing. 2015:13,174.

Osler Symposium. Sir William Osler and his inspirational words. [Internet]. 2016. Available at: http://www.oslersymposia.org/about-Sir-William-Osler.html. Accessed June 9, 2016.

Remens RN. Healer's art. [Internet]. 2012. Available at: http://www.rachelremen.com/learn/medical-education-work/. Accessed June 8, 2016.

Shapiro J. Forgiving ourselves for being human: normalizing the isolating experience of adverse events. [Internet]. 2014. Available at: http://www.gold-foundation.org/forgiving-human-normalizing-isolating-experience-adverse-events/. Accessed June 9, 2016.

Shapiro J, Galowitz P. Peer support for clinicians: a programmatic approach. *Acad Med.* 2016;91(9).

West CP, Dyrbye LN, Rabatin JT, et al. Intervention to promote physician well-being, job satisfaction, and professionalism: a randomized clinical trial. *JAMA Intern Med.* 2014;174(4):527–533.

# CHAPTER 10

## DISMANTLING THE WORKPLACE DRIVERS OF BURNOUT

*Being continually poked with a sharp stick is what
leads to burnout. It's the extra stuff that interferes, like
EHR work, paperwork, transit time. To fix burnout,
we need to identify and get rid of the "pokes."*
—MONTGOMERY ELMER, MD, FAMILY
MEDICINE PHYSICIAN AT THEDACARE

*Health care leaders are spanning profound sheering forces
of "Make your health care delivery system better or else."
They often respond by mandating, dictating, and pressuring
physicians. This makes physicians feel without control and
without connection to the very essence of what it means
to be a physician. It disconnects them from the positive
behaviors that would allow these changes to manifest.*
—STEPHEN BEESON, MD, PHYSICIAN, AUTHOR, AND
FOUNDER OF THE PHYSICIAN EFFECTIVENESS PROJECT

Health care organizations across the country have acknowledged the problem of physician burnout. In our experience, the most common responses have been educating clinicians about burnout and instituting wellness programs to build resiliency. Although these are important steps, they do not address the frustrations and barriers in the clinical workplace that are the true sources of the problem. To prevent physician burnout—and fix these underlying problems that affect other performance metrics—organizations need to adopt other solutions.

Some forward-thinking organizations have looked beyond wellness initiatives to address the workplace drivers of burnout. In this chapter, we'll highlight some of these organizations and their innovative interventions.

## MISSION HEALTH: COMMUNICATING WITH THE FRONT LINES

Headquartered in Asheville, North Carolina, Mission Health is a large, integrated health system with a medical staff of more than 1,000 physicians. Ronald A. Paulus, MD, president and CEO of the organization, launched an initiative to improve communication between the C-suite and frontline clinicians using an innovative digital platform.

WikiWisdom was designed by a former election pollster to gather responses to specific questions. It's anonymous and monitored by a third-party moderator. A series of questions are posed, and participants voice their opinions about problems and potential solutions. The moderator identifies the most vocal thought leaders and coordinates their input to create a written report, which a small group presents to Paulus in a face-to-face meeting.

The CEO has used information captured in the WikiWisdom reports to make rapid fixes to problems that had plagued the frontline staff, but were never communicated all the way up the chain of command.

For example, through the nurses' WikiWisdom report, he learned that for years seasoned nurses had objected to having to take the personality test given to new hires when they transferred from one job to another within the system. One week later the requirement was eliminated.

Via the physicians' WikiWisdom report, Paulus came to appreciate "the hassle factor"—the daily frustrations and barriers to patient care that were burning out physicians. Chief among these was the EHR. According to Paulus, the report made the problem "real and tangible."

He presented a proposal to the Mission Health board for a program to improve the usability of the EHR and fix inefficient workflow processes. Board members were well informed about the daily lives of clinicians at the organization through a separate initiative called Immersion Day. During Immersion Day, board members and local policy makers don scrubs, sign privacy forms, and spend 9 to 12 hours behind the scenes, watching frontline clinicians in their everyday work and gaining insights they could never have acquired otherwise.

Despite the multimillion-dollar price tag, the board unanimously agreed to fund the clinician well-being and EHR optimization program. Board members had seen firsthand the reality of daily practice and were convinced of the necessity of the investment to fix the workplace problems. The program provides funding for several initiatives, including dedicated IT specialists (five FTEs' worth) to shadow physicians and identify specific problems in the EHR software. The shadowing aspect is essential, Paulus told us, because finding specific problems is a challenge. "You can't crack the surface with the EHR problems, because people don't remember or can't describe the problem scenario. The IT shadow can observe and ask pertinent questions of the clinician, and he or she can say, 'I get insane from this,' and point out the issue. Then the problem is actionable."

Paulus told us, "WikiWisdom is a very effective, low-cost, easy, rapid way to get direct visualization on what's going on in the minds of the people who really matter." The initiative provides valuable information to leaders, and it models respect for the frontline doctors and nurses. The feedback from frontline physicians also led Paulus to become more involved on a national level in advocating for solutions to physician burnout.

## UMHS PRIMARY CARE CLINIC: FIXING FRUSTRATIONS AT THE FRONT LINES

University of Michigan Health System (UMHS), a large, academic medical center located in Ann Arbor, employs about 25,000 workers. John E. "Jack" Billi, MD, has been a general internist in a primary care clinic at UMHS for 38 years. A decade ago he was tapped to become a senior Lean deployment leader at the health system. A significant focus of his work has been helping frontline workers acquire the skills they need to find and fix the root causes of the problems they face every day.

Frontline teams and improvement specialists worked together in rapid improvement events (RIEs) to create the health system's "Lean in Daily Work" model, which is a framework for operationalizing Lean at the front lines. To date, the model has been spread to more than 75 percent of the 150 clinics at the medical center. It includes teaching and implementing the philosophy and components of Lean (which we'll describe in detail in the next chapter). The model creates a process and structure through which frontline workers (both clinical and non-clinical) identify current and potential problems and take responsibility for suggesting and trying possible solutions. Managers provide needed support and resources to experiment with the proposed fix and ensure that the various tests of change don't conflict with each other.

To encourage physicians to engage fully in the work, Billi reminds them that they are already comfortable with the scientific method as it's applied to patient care. Lean is the application of the same method to the processes of care. To engage physicians who are initially resistant to Lean, Billi ensures that the group addresses problems that affect physicians as well. He tells physicians, "Lean will turn you from victims of burnout to people who have the power to change things."

In an interview, Billi shared a three-part process he uses to engage physicians in Lean.

- Motive: This step ensures that physicians see improvement as part of their job and that they believe they can succeed in improvement initiatives.
- Means: This part entails teaching physicians to analyze their work and use a scientific process to identify and fix workplace problems.
- Opportunity: In this step, Billi helps physicians see that investing the time to understand and fix work processes is valuable because it puts them in an empowered position from which they can improve processes and patient care. He also ensures that a system is in place that provides physicians with dedicated time to talk about improvements. One example of a way to ensure such dedicated time is to close the clinic for an hour each week.

In an interview, Billi used an allegory to explain the importance of fixing workplace problems. A group of clinicians is picnicking by a river when a body floats by. Several clinicians pull the person out of the flow and start CPR. A second body floats by, and the clinicians pull out this person and start resuscitation procedures. A third body and then a fourth and a fifth float by. The clinicians are beginning to get overwhelmed trying to keep up with the continual flow of people needing help. Billi pointed out, "No one thinks to go upstream and find out what is causing the people to fall in the river in the first place." He completed the story by drawing the analogy to broken workplace processes, saying, "Physicians are flogged by the daily crush, but they need to stop what they're doing and go upstream to figure out the cause of these problems. Otherwise, they will be condemned to be victims of the broken processes forever."

Billi has found that the most significant obstacle to physician engagement in Lean is their belief that organizational leaders don't care about the daily circumstances at the front lines of care. "If senior leaders don't feel their pain, physicians lose confidence. Leaders need to go to the front lines, see what's going on, ask questions, and show respect." Another important obstacle is physicians becoming overwhelmed by the size and scope of a problem. He encourages physicians to break the issue into small, clear, actionable problems, and then start with one small problem. For example, instead of trying to tackle increasing access to care for all pediatric patients, focus first on a more manageable target: reducing the length of time for a return visit in the pediatric hematology clinic. He also reminds physicians to expect failure for many of their initial tests of change, because finding effective solutions is often an iterative process.

## OREGON MEDICAL GROUP: ENABLING PHYSICIAN LEADERSHIP

Oregon Medical Group is an independent, physician-led, 135-provider, multispecialty group located in the Eugene, Oregon, area. According to Karen Weiner, MD, a pediatrician and chief medical officer of the practice, when she was serving on the board several years ago, she saw that physician burnout was a substantial barrier to achieving their organizational goals. She told us that the effects of health care reform and the onslaught of new mandates had brought physicians' morale to an all-time low. The suicide of a pediatrician colleague brought home the urgency of the problem.

In 2013, Weiner was promoted to medical director, a full-time position created to address low physician satisfaction and morale. Her first step was to use the MBI to measure the prevalence of burnout among her colleagues. Weiner used the results as a burning platform to make the case that changes were needed across the organization. "The results were a wake-up call for our doctors that we had to do something differently," she told us.

The group supported Weiner's leadership training; she completed a master's degree in medical management to better understand how to develop a physician-supportive organization. For the capstone project of her degree program, she developed a methodology for teaching other health care leaders about organizational burnout—how to assess, address, and ultimately prevent it through effective leadership and culture.

Weiner's project has been instructive on many levels. She has learned about the important role of leadership in preventing burnout. As she put it, "Most executives don't know what burnout is or how to prevent it. Leaders must understand burnout and the organizational factors that contribute to burnout. Some of the key factors are control, fairness, rewards, and values." She's learned about the connection between lack of control and burnout. "Some physicians have preconceived ideas of the causes of burnout and don't think it can change. They get stuck in eddies and stop thinking about solutions, because they feel they have no control."

Weiner has also developed a deeper understanding of disruptive physician behavior. She cites a joint RAND/American Medical Association study that identified perceived barriers to providing quality care as the number one source of dissatisfaction among physicians. (Friedberg 2013) As she put it, "Inappropriate responses or angry yelling happen because the physician feels unable to provide the quality of care they want. One of the greatest contributors to burnout is doing work that doesn't honor your personal values or feeling that your values are not honored in your daily work."

Weiner sees physician burnout as a signal of underlying organizational issues. "If the leader of an organization has a lot of dissatisfied physicians, it's showing that the physicians are perceiving barriers to providing quality care. It's a strong indicator that something's wrong."

Weiner believes that interventions are needed at four levels—individual, professional, organizational, and societal—to address physician burnout. She tries to keep leaders of her physician group focused on the organization-level interventions. "Mindfulness and other individual solutions are a great resource, but if you only give physicians these solutions, it's like saying, 'If you only knew how to swim better, this toxic ocean wouldn't be a problem.' Getting sidetracked on the individual solutions can prevent leaders from doing anything about the organizational interventions."

Weiner believes that one of the most important organization-level interventions to help address physician burnout is increasing the number of physician leaders: "Filling in the depth and breadth of physician leadership is a must. I'm very concerned to see some organizations are cutting back on education for developing physician leaders."

The practice group began expanding physician leadership by providing physicians with a view of the future state of the organization and enabling them to collaboratively create a shared vision based on that future state. Leaders and physicians worked together to craft and individually sign a compact that outlines the responsibilities of the organization and the physicians to each other. The compact also delineated new rules of engagement. Once this foundation work was completed, leaders worked with physicians to redesign many aspects of operations and clarified physicians' roles in improvement projects, specifically ensuring that all projects had clear end points. Subsequently, physicians' participation in improvement projects increased dramatically. The group has begun to implement Lean, with a focus on removing waste as a barrier to patient care and on maximizing the impact of physicians' work.

Participation in successful improvement projects has fostered greater interest among physicians in taking leadership roles. Over the course of about two years, the group has undergone a significant culture change. Weiner says, "We now have a collaborative culture within our group. There is a sense of excitement and momentum in the work now." For the past several years, the group has measured physician burnout, anonymously by department, using the Maslach Burnout Inventory (MBI). Because the MBI provides prevalence rates but does not indicate causes, the group also implements the American Medical Group Association's physician satisfaction survey to identify problematic areas. If a department has high burnout scores, Weiner meets with the physicians as a group and one-on-one to identify the specific causes of burnout. Since the increased attention to physician leadership and implementation of fixes to specific workplace issues, the group's average physician burnout score for emotional exhaustion (EE) has dropped from 27.7 to 23.1, well below the threshold of "high degree of burnout," which is defined as an EE score of 27.

Although these improvements stem from many interventions, a primary one, according to Weiner, is the expansion of physician leadership.

## MEDICAL ASSOCIATES CLINIC AND HEALTH PLANS: IMPROVING PHYSICIANS' DAILY WORK

Medical Associates Clinic and Health Plans is a 170-provider, multispecialty group practice in Dubuque, Iowa. Several years ago, Christine Sinsky, MD, a general internist at the medical group and vice president of professional satisfaction at the American Medical Association, realized that she needed to change the way she was practicing if she was going to continue. She had come face-to-face with a disquieting realization: "What the patient valued and what I valued were the same, but that was not where I was spending my time."

That realization, combined with the desire to stay in clinical practice, led to a sweeping change in the way she and her team deliver care. The practice shifted to a team-based model and focused on removing the daily frustrations that had caused significant stress. Each physician, working in a team with nurses and medical assistants, shares the responsibilities of patient care. By working in concert with other clinical staff within a team, physicians are able to focus on doing the tasks that only physicians can do, which means more time in direct patient care.

When creating the standard care processes, clinicians identified and eliminated the root problems that caused frustrations and inefficiencies.

This effort ultimately resulted in streamlined care processes and improved care coordination. In an interview, Sinsky said, "We standardized the predictable aspects of work to be the default. The standard processes allow physicians to spend most of their time on the 15 percent that falls outside the routine."

The clinicians created pre-visit and post-visit processes that have made the total care processes much more consistent and reliable. For example, a nurse completes pre-visit planning two or three days before a scheduled patient visit, reviewing previous notes, ensuring that any lab results are available, identifying preventive and chronic care needs, and reminding patients of their visit.

A specific intervention the practice instituted to improve physicians' daily work is revamping the role of nurses. At the beginning of a visit, the nurse prescreens the patient, updating the medical record, reconciling medications, completing an initial history, and identifying the patient's chief objectives for the visit. During the physician portion of the visit, the nurse helps document and retrieve information from the EHR, which enables the physician to focus his or her full attention on the patient. At the conclusion of the visit, the nurse arranges follow-up visits, submits requests for referrals and tests, and ensures the patient understands the care plan. Because the nurse has been involved during the visit, he or she is more knowledgeable about the care plan and can more effectively coordinate between-visit care. The connection also enhances the relationship between the nurse and each patient.

Members of the care team hold a short (no more than 15 minutes) huddle each morning. During the huddle, the team ensures that staff and resources are sufficient for the day and that all team members are aware of any potential issues. Care team members sit in close proximity to each other to facilitate communication and reduce delays in completing tasks that require an information exchange. As a result of the close communication afforded by the team-based model, Sinsky and her colleagues have found that their inboxes are not filled with messages at the end of the work day, because other team members have already responded to them.

Team-based care has changed the practice from being reactive to being proactive, fostering a greater sense of control over the work environment. It has also fostered greater accountability among all the staff for care quality and the patient experience. Sinsky told us, "We've instituted changes to make the practice a single unit from which the patient receives care. Now, when our staff are referring to patients they say, 'my patient,' rather than, 'Dr. Sinsky's patient.' On the phone, they now ask, 'What can I do for you?'" The model has changed the culture of the practice for everyone. Sinsky said, "We are better able to connect with our patients and practice has become fun again."

## HENNEPIN COUNTY MEDICAL CENTER: FOSTERING IMPROVED WORK-LIFE BALANCE

Located in Minneapolis, Minnesota, Hennepin County Medical Center (HCMC) is an academic, safety net health system with more than 6,800 physicians and clinical staff. Mark Linzer, MD, a general internist at HCMC and a researcher on physician burnout, told us that giving physicians more control over their work has been important in addressing burnout at the health system. By doing so, the organization has taken steps to address two key drivers of burnout: lack of control and work-life imbalance.

In the past, the organization had held strict policies about the timing of patient's visits in the outpatient clinics. Linzer noted that the policy often caused significant stress for physicians who were the parents of young children. When the clinic ran late or a patient with a complication arrived just before closing, the physicians were pressed for time to drive across town in rush-hour traffic to pick up a child from daycare on time. "It was a recipe for burnout," Linzer said.

For many years Linzer's team has conducted surveys to monitor the burnout level of physicians in different divisions at HCMC. The team presented administration with data showing a high burnout rate among physicians in the clinic and worked with administration to change the policy to allow for a more flexible schedule. If desired, physicians can now elect to start and end their clinic hours earlier. "Rather than burning out and leaving practice," Linzer said, "These physicians have stayed, in part because they were given greater control over their daily schedule."

Linzer has been especially cognizant of the need to improve work-life balance for parent-clinicians. The health system has offered several solutions to address their needs, including flexible schedules, on-site childcare, part-time practice, and shared positions. In presentations, Linzer often relays an experience that exemplifies the organization's culture and its efforts to support physicians with young children. One afternoon, Linzer and an administrator were meeting in the general medicine clinic on a day when Linzer was not scheduled to see patients. In passing, one of the physicians told them that she was hosting a party that evening for her daughter's third birthday. Linzer and the administrator canceled their meeting and Linzer took over her remaining visits, allowing her to go home early.

In his presentations, Linzer shows the thank-you card he later received, with a photograph of the girl blowing out her birthday candles and the message, "Dear Dr. Mark, thank you for helping out my mom..." He makes the point that everyone, physicians included, goes through many life events for which support is helpful: pregnancy, parenting young children, caring for sick or elderly relatives, or the death of a loved one or friend. He encourages the leaders of clinical departments to offer flexible work arrangements and plan coverage for these events to avoid overburdening physicians.

To advance work-life balance across the health system, Linzer and his team launched an Office of Professional Worklife (OPW) in 2014. The space is a visible site for clinician wellness, with a "reset room" where clinicians can find a quiet respite for a few moments in their work day. The OPW team conducts annual surveys of stress and burnout, collaborates with the health system's provider wellness committee, and works with departments within HCMC to develop action-oriented plans to address burnout, based on the specific issues in each practice area. Within the year following the OPW opening, burnout rates dropped by 20 percent. Linzer and his team continue to look for ways to improve work-life balance for physicians in the organization and, through their research, for physicians across the country.

As Linzer summed up in a 2011 presentation to medical staff at Stanford, "[To prevent burnout], it's always tempting to try and remove demands, but good luck trying to do that. [Instead], give people control of the work environment, give them support, and all of a sudden they are back in balance. It's not easy, but it can be done." (Stanford 2011)

## WALNUT HILL MEDICAL CENTER: ENABLING A PHYSICIAN-LED VISION

Located in Dallas, Walnut Hill Medical Center (WHMC) is a 100-bed hospital designed by physicians to optimize care delivery for patients and care providers. Ricardo Guerra, Jr., MD, a practicing cardiologist and executive board member at the organization, explained that the founding physicians persevered during the 10 years from inspiration to the ribbon-cutting ceremony in April 2014, because they wanted to practice in a health care organization with strong physician leadership and a positive organizational culture.

According to Guerra, opening the hospital was a way for physicians to take back the control of patient care in the face of substantial changes in the health care environment. The organization is managed and governed by physicians, and four physicians sit on the seven-member board of directors. Guerra says, "From the beginning, we thought about how to optimize the physician's experience because it's right for physicians and it works." Maintaining a strong physician presence in leadership is a core value of the organization. As Guerra described it, "Non-clinical leaders are not going to have the same orientation as physician leaders; physician leaders are naturally geared to thinking about what's best for the patient."

The culture of WHMC is illustrated by a statement on its website: "Walnut Hill Medical Center is not just a brand-new hospital. It's a new approach to the patient and caregiver experience...We do what it takes to make sure every patient receives the personalized, compassionate care he or she deserves. We give our caregivers the support they need to make patient care their top priority." (WHMC website) The organization has used a proactive strategy to create and maintain a positive culture.

One component of the strategy was looking outside of health care for lessons on building an exceptional service organization. Leaders reviewed the practices of companies that were known for exceptional customer service, such as Apple and Ritz Carlton. From these ideas the leaders built the corporate practices, which have shaped the organizational culture. "We adopted the belief that happy employees lead to happy customers. If we take care of our staff, they will take care of our patients," said Guerra.

Employee hiring is one example of how WHMC's culture has been shaped by corporate practices. According to Guerra, leaders believe that job-related tasks can be taught but that caring cannot. Because a caring culture is a top priority, the organization selects potential hires for their aptitude for service, based on questions that assess caring and aptitude for working on a team.

All new employees attend an orientation presentation by Guerra in which he introduces them to the expectations for behavior and attitude. At the orientation he tells them, "We chose you because we believe you can help us with our vision. We want you to come to work to make a difference in people's lives and do it by being kind." He explained to us that the organization's positive culture has spread by word of mouth among job seekers, such that the vacancy rate for positions is low. The organization accepts just 3 percent of all job applicants.

Training policies are another example of the influence of the organization's corporate practices on culture. Employees receive specific training for communicating and interacting with patients; the steps of such communication and interaction, given in the following list, form the acronym WE CARE:

- **W**arm welcome and personalized greeting
- **E**mpathize
- **C**ommunicate and connect
- **A**ddress the patient's concerns, questions, and needs, both expressed and unexpressed
- **R**esolve and reassure
- **E**nd with a fond farewell

Guerra explained that WE CARE is more than a customer service program: it is the basis for the organization's culture.

Frontline problem-solving with the rapid addressing of issues was also a component of the culture-building strategy. To engage clinical staff and physicians in problem-solving, the organization created a WE CARE committee. This group brings frontline staff together to identify problems related to patient flow, equipment, and access and to brainstorm potential solutions. "Because the meetings include representatives from other relevant units, the group can quickly talk through solutions, and how to measure success, and create a proposal," Guerra told us.

"Through the process, the frontline clinicians now have a voice and can have an impact on issues that affect them."

Hiring a chief experience officer (CXO) was another proactive step the organization took to optimize culture. Guerra pointed out the importance of having a senior leader responsible for the overall care experience, because he or she can cross the departmental silos that exist in an organization. He said, "The CXO is like the conductor of a symphony. You have many highly skilled individuals each focused on one role. The conductor helps them work together to create an excellent performance. The CXO is the agent for culture development and maintenance."

According to Guerra, the positive culture at WHMC helps prevent burnout by helping people find meaning in their work. "Burnout is one of the reasons we wanted to do something different when we conceived of our hospital 10 years ago. We aim to create a culture that gives people meaning. We try to reconnect physicians and other caregivers with the higher goal of improving people's lives."

The results? WHMC has achieved 99th percentile scores for patient satisfaction. The organization also recently set about to improve IT for physicians. After hiring a new CIO to address the EHR inefficiencies, the organization received a HIMSS Level 6 designation, placing it in the top quartile nationally, according to Guerra.

## ADVENTIST HEALTH SYSTEM: PRIORITIZING PHYSICIAN WELL-BEING

Adventist Health System (AHS) is a 46-hospital, integrated system headquartered in Altamonte Springs, Florida. According to Ted Hamilton, MD, vice president for medical mission at the organization, a dozen years ago leaders realized that although they had actively engaged staff in the mission, they had not been intentional about engaging physicians in mission-based work. At that point, Hamilton told us, the CEO realized, "'To engage physicians, we need to do something for them.' We didn't know the word for burnout then." Hamilton was asked to lead initiatives to support physician well-being and engagement and to collaborate with other organizations to combat burnout.

Hamilton launched Physician Support Services (PSS) at Florida Hospital, AHS's 2,000-bed flagship hospital. PSS is an employee assistance program specifically for physicians. The organization hired a psychologist to shadow physicians to better understand their work stressors. She then interviewed physicians at the hospital, and she continues to interview new doctors as they come on staff so that she can get a sense of their background and personal circumstances and can inform them of the availability of counseling. To date, the program has offered more than 10,000 counseling visits.

In 2010, Hamilton joined with leaders of other three other health systems to found the Coalition for Physician Well-Being, for which he currently serves as chair of the executive committee. The coalition now represents 20 health care organizations that are committed to combatting physician burnout. The group convenes an annual meeting and holds monthly webinars on topics such as depression, burnout, and values. Hamilton told us, "At the coalition's annual meeting, physicians talk about work, stress, rest, marriage—their personal lives. They tell us they are amazed and grateful that a health care system cares enough about their welfare to convene the program." The two-day meeting includes plenary sessions, smaller break-out activities, and table discussions. Topics presented in the past include purpose and meaning, marriage and family, spirituality, and service.

The commitment of AHS leaders to these initiatives demonstrates a deep respect for physicians as humans and a profound understanding that physicians' well-being is critical to compassionate health care and to fulfilling the spiritual mission of the organization.

## VANCOUVER CLINIC: ENGAGING PHYSICIANS IN STRATEGY DEVELOPMENT

Located in Washington State across the Columbia River from Portland, Oregon, the Vancouver Clinic is a multispecialty medical group with about 250 care providers. Despite the fact that the organization is owned and governed by physicians, leaders saw increasing dissatisfaction and a growing lack of engagement among physicians. According to Sharon A. Crowell, MD, an internist and chair of the board of Vancouver Clinic, they received comments such as, "Over the past 10 years there has been a steady deterioration in the physicians' influence over the operations of the clinic...Every major decision is heavily influenced by non physician administrators...This has led to a clinic that is very much top-down oriented." The practice scored an abysmal 11th percentile on a national survey of provider satisfaction.

The drop in satisfaction followed an intense focus by the CEO on infrastructure and finance after a downturn in the economy and a constriction of the market. According to Alfred H. Seekamp, MD, obstetrician and chief medical officer of the organization, when the CEO announced his retirement in 2011, leaders and the board feared that the incoming executive leader was doomed to fail unless the existing gulf between the administration and physicians was resolved. Seekamp was concerned about burnout from an individual and an organizational perspective. "Burnout can be a disaster in an organization where you need engagement."

To ensure that the organization could achieve its mission and goals, leaders fully engaged frontline providers in the development of the group's strategy. They also adopted a new approach to leadership— one that was grounded in respect and bidirectional communication. In January 2012, organizational leaders implemented the nominal-group technique to better understand physicians' work experiences. They convened informal focus groups of physicians and asked them to describe their daily frontline experience at the clinic. At a dinner meeting, a group facilitator asked two simple questions: What would make your life at Vancouver Clinic rich and meaningful? What's getting in the way?

Physicians wrote their responses to the questions on index cards, engaged in short table conversations to identify broad themes, and presented a summary to the group. According to Crowell, the process generated extremely valuable data. She explained, "In two and a half hours, we had hundreds of individual comments, from which we developed a list of themes that reflected the physicians' hopes and dreams. We brought that information into a leadership retreat and used it to guide the creation of our new strategic vision." After the retreat, leaders shared the written vision at the organization's monthly meeting to confirm its accuracy and to demonstrate that the physicians' input was valued. "The process was so successful that we use it for every big decision now," Crowell told us.

Seekamp explained that the iterative technique used in the new strategic planning process was key to re-engaging physicians. "The process works as an engagement spiral. We show physicians that they have the ability to influence leadership, which leads to trust. Trust leads to engagement." The planning process also identified key pain points that were affecting the physicians' daily work experience. Department chairs followed up by asking physicians about specific problem areas and potential solutions. The interventions were included in the organization's strategic plan. For example, pediatricians wanted to maintain continuity with their panel of patients, but when a provider had a full day's schedule, patients with acute issues would be scheduled for a same-day appointment with another care provider, which then limited same-day appointments for his or her own patients. As a solution, the group now schedules patients with their assigned care provider on another day or triages them to the urgent care clinic. The organization is also testing the use of medical scribes to alleviate the data-entry burden identified by physicians.

Vancouver Clinic also adopted a daily management system to improve communication across the organization. Seekamp believes it may help prevent burnout. "The management system allows clinicians to be more effective at their work and helps alleviate the sense of being overwhelmed and burned out. Plus, it engages both physicians and staff."

Seekamp and Crowell described the improvement in culture and physician engagement at the organization. A recent survey showed that physician satisfaction scores had risen to the 75th percentile. According to Crowell, there is a perceptible increase in physicians' joy in practice. "Once physicians see they can influence leadership, they readily engage in solving problems to improve their work environment." Other metrics support her observations: provider turnover has decreased, recruitment of new physicians has become easier, and physicians' productivity, as measured by RVUs per FTE, has increased.

Seekamp summed up the shift in strategic planning this way: "This process is not top-down decision-making. It is understanding what's working well and where problems exist in the organization by asking appropriate questions. Leaders don't solve the problems for people. Instead we help them find and implement solutions."

## NORTHEAST GEORGIA PHYSICIANS GROUP: ELIMINATING DAILY FRUSTRATIONS IN THE PRIMARY CARE SETTING

Northeast Georgia Physicians Group (NGPG) is a large, multispecialty group with more than 50 locations in northern Georgia. One clinic, located in the small town of Cleveland, served as a model site for the group's Lean implementation. Providers at the primary care clinic include three physicians and a nurse practitioner. According to James Murphey, MD, an internist and pediatrician at the clinic, one of the most pressing problems for care providers there was the daily struggle—and failure—to keep on schedule. It was not unusual for patients to wait an hour or more to see their care provider. Murphey told us, "I was struggling with being behind all day. There was a snowball effect, with longer and longer delays as the day went on and no chance to catch up. It was stressful for providers and patients."

After identifying inefficiencies in their daily work through rapid improvement events (RIEs), the clinicians and staff made a number of changes. Staff adapted the schedule to account for triage time and for appointment duration. They also included time in the schedule for documentation. The clinicians and staff standardized certain processes to streamline the workflow.

Murphey admitted to feeling wary about standardization when the idea was first introduced. He said, "A lot of providers shy away from standardization when they hear about it. A year ago I would have felt the same way." Murphey told us that what sold him was learning about Lean principles and seeing the processes at work during a study trip in which he observed a clinic that had implemented Lean. "I really needed to see it for myself to believe," he said.

What Murphey and the other care providers at the clinic have found is that standardizing the operational aspects of the patient visit has freed up time to deal with the variability that inevitably arises. As he put it, "By controlling all that we can, we can deal with the unknown better." Murphey feels the changes have allowed him to practice medicine the way he had hoped to when he entered the profession. "My time with patients has not changed, but the rest of the office processes and operations around that time have changed. The improvements have preserved the kind of medicine we want to practice."

According to Murphey, all the providers experienced benefits from the practice changes, although the degree to which they were affected varied. He told us, "One provider was already very efficient with documentation. It took several RIEs before he noticed changes, like staying on time with his scheduled appointments, less staff overtime, and improved morale." Murphey noticed changes immediately, with a substantial reduction in his "after-hours" documentation work.

Physicians at the clinic had expected their productivity to decline with the new processes, especially with the time set aside in the schedule for documentation. However, following an initial dip during the first few months after launching the Lean implementation, the physicians' productivity has increased 10 percent over baseline. Additionally, the number of appointments starting on time has doubled, and the average time a patient spends in the clinic per appointment has decreased from 80 minutes to 45 minutes.

Murphey sees the practice changes that the group instituted as being essential for avoiding burnout and for continuing to practice over the long haul. Although he was just six years out of training, before the Lean implementation Murphey questioned whether he could keep up the pace, especially with the way work was impinging on his home life. "I don't know how long I could have continued to work as I was. Now I have time for more of a life—to exercise and spend with family. It has made my life more balanced. Now I can see myself practicing for 20 or 30 years."

The three final vignettes describe organizations that have maintained a consistent commitment to Lean transformation across their entire organization.

## THEDACARE: PIONEERING LEAN IN HEALTH CARE BY FOCUSING ON LEAN PRINCIPLES

ThedaCare, a mid-sized health care system located in the Fox Valley of central Wisconsin, comprises multiple hospitals, physicians' offices, and ancillary support services. Prior to 2002, the health care system had consistently performed well in national quality of care rankings, due in large part to a long history of dedication to quality and service. However, maintaining that quality level required heroic efforts by many of the physicians and leaders.

In 2002, two years into his tenure as CEO, John Toussaint, MD, began to look for a better way to run the system. One of the members of his board of directors owned and ran a business that manufactured snowblowers; the company used the Toyota Production System to manage its operations.

ThedaCare leaders visited the snowblower factory to learn the principles of Lean production. They engaged Lean coaches to guide them through the process of adapting Lean manufacturing to health care. With the assistance of the coaches, ThedaCare leaders simplified what they learned into fundamental principles that were based on Continuous Improvement and Respect for People; these principles were focusing on patients, identifying value from the patient's perspective, and minimizing the time required for a course of treatment.

The resulting ThedaCare Improvement System included all the key elements of fully deployed Lean. The organization identified True North Metrics (TNMs), which leaders monitor to ensure everyone at the organization maintains a focus on the most important aspects of their work. Leaders and managers track performance on TNMs visually on boards throughout the hospital, from frontline patient care areas to the boardroom. Leaders use the TNMs in their Strategy Deployment process to provide focus. They also use the TNMs to decide which initiatives to "de-select," in order to avoid overloading frontline staff and managers and their focus on the most important priorities.

Based on Lean management processes in manufacturing, ThedaCare developed a new approach to managing the business of health care. Leaders developed a Daily Management System that supports operations on the front lines and connects the front lines with the C-suite through a system of tiered daily huddles. In the frontline huddles, staff members and their managers identify and solve problems. Any problems that cannot be solved at the local level are escalated, all the way to the CEO if necessary, to the level at which they can be solved within a single day.

The organization uses Value Stream Mapping (VSM) to effect major redesign of specific care processes. During VSM, a team of staff and managers tracks the flow of the patient from the beginning to the end of the process, identifying wasteful steps and processes along the way. Using this approach throughout its clinical settings, the organization pioneered collaborative care team models for inpatient and outpatient work, including life-saving care for patients with heart attacks and strokes.

Realizing the challenge of spreading Lean thinking and processes across an entity as diverse and complex as a health system, leaders created a Lean Promotion Office to develop internal expertise in Lean and to guide managers through personal development to become a Lean leader. Leaders also addressed succession planning, a key factor in ensuring long-term commitment to Lean as a management system, so that when Toussaint retired from his position as CEO, his replacement would carry on the work. In fact, ThedaCare's Lean approach continues to this day, years after Toussaint's departure.

How does ThedaCare's experience apply to burnout? Lean transformation substantially changed the work life of everyone at ThedaCare. Toussaint told us about a hypothesis he formed early in his work as CEO of the organization. "We believed that creating stability in work processes would lead to better work-life balance for providers and better outcomes for patients. Over time, we proved this was true. I'm often stopped on the street by physicians and nurses who say, 'Thank you for bringing us a different way of thinking,' because it stabilized their lives." Physicians have told him that they would have cut back their workloads or retired early were it not for Lean.

## DENVER HEALTH: ENGAGING PHYSICIANS THROUGH ENGAGED LEADERSHIP

Denver Health is a public, academic, integrated health system that serves about one-third of the residents of Denver. The safety net hospital faced escalating financial stress as economic shifts increased the number of uninsured—who make up about one-third of the organization's patients—and decreased reimbursement.

In 2005, the organization began its Lean transformation journey, eventually reaping a range of positive outcomes. For example, the organization had the lowest risk-adjusted trauma mortality rate for level 1 trauma centers in the state in the 2007–2009 data period—with a mortality ratio 26 percent below that expected for a hospital with its case mix. (Gabow 2011) The number of sentinel events decreased from 13 in 2008 to 2 in 2010. (Gabow 2011) Between July 2006 and December 2012, the organization saw a financial benefit (that is, money saved and increased revenue) of about $195 million by removing waste and inefficiencies. (Gabow 2015) More recently, the organization used Lean tools to transform primary care clinics to the patient-centered medical home model, with all staff working at the top of their licenses. In less than three years, all clinics were certified at level 1 or 2 under the new NCQA certification (Paul Melinkovich, MD, personal communication, January 28, 2016). Deep involvement of leadership has been an essential element in the organization's success.

When introducing Lean to Denver Health staff in 2004, CEO Patricia A. Gabow, MD, emphasized the importance of the transformation in protecting the organization's deeply held mission to maintain access to high-quality care for everyone, regardless of ability to pay. At the annual CEO address she told them, "Denver Health is going to take the road less traveled. We have only three options when faced with increased uninsured patients and decreased revenues: cut services to the uninsured, increase revenues, or dramatically improve efficiency. We're going to maintain our mission and select the third." (Hafer 2012)

She also prioritized equity. "Everyone was treated the same," she told us in an interview. "I had the same vacation time as the housekeepers." She acknowledged positive contributions to the organization by staff at every level. She relayed that at an annual, standing-room-only State of Denver Health address, she presented the CEO award to a member of the grounds crew who had exemplified dedication to improving the patient experience. He received a standing ovation from the staff and leaders. "Everyone found meaning in the work we were doing. Everyone's work was appreciated," she said. In fact, the Lean Black Belts, a cadre of about 250 staff members with training in Lean, were initially provided with small financial rewards for the savings they achieved. "They didn't want it, because it decreased collaboration between units," she told us.

Gabow also emphasized transparency and fairness, ensuring that leaders were as involved as frontline staff in improvement work. She found that being a physician herself proved advantageous when working with frontline physicians. "I could tell them what needed to be done and they could hear me. In turn, they couldn't pull the wool over my eyes about what was possible or not possible. I could speak their language." According to Rick Dart, formerly at Denver Health, Gabow's ability to speak directly to physicians changed their level of engagement in improvement: "Before the mid-1990s physicians' [attitudes were] not ideal. Many had a chip on their shoulders, having come to Denver Health because of the mission to help the poor. They were basically saying, 'I'll do what I want. You're lucky to have me here.'"

According to Paul Melinkovich of Denver Health, Gabow and other leaders used several techniques to improve physician engagement in improvement. He said, "It's important for leaders to help physicians understand that Lean is not a top-down endeavor and to recognize that the primary goal is not to improve finances, though it may. Instead, they need to appeal to higher ideals, like quality, safety, and the patient experience."

## SUTTER GOULD MEDICAL FOUNDATION: DEVELOPING LEADERSHIP DYADS ACROSS THE ENTERPRISE

"Everywhere I went, the doctors and staff were happy." When we interviewed Steven Mitnick, MD, CMO of Sutter Gould Medical Foundation and Gould Medical Group ("Gould"), he shared with us this quote from a surveyor at the conclusion of a recent accreditation survey. Mitnick told us that the surveyor was surprised and said that finding happy physicians and staff was unusual at busy medical groups.

Gould launched its Lean journey in 2009. Two weeks after Paul DeChant, MD, became the CEO of the foundation, he attended an American Medical Group Association (AGMA) meeting in which ThedaCare leaders described their approach to redesigning primary care clinics. He saw the potential to do the same at Gould. Fortunately, Mitnick was looking for just such an opportunity. Together, they spoke with the leaders at ThedaCare, chose Simpler as their consulting group, and launched Gould's Lean transformation with the theme of "Returning Joy to Patient Care."

Gould Medical Group was founded 60 years ago by two brothers who had graduated from the Mayo Clinic and wanted to create a Mayo-model, multispecialty medical group in California's Central Valley. The group was converted to a foundation model in the 1980s and joined Sutter Health in the 1990s. The organization grew steadily over the years to become a 300-physician group. It included 23 specialties with 1,100 support staff working in 25 locations spread over a 50-mile swath of some of the most productive farmland in the country.

When assumed the CEO position at the foundation, the medical group had just completed a process to redefine their vision statement. They defined it as: "The Gould Medical Group will be nationally recognized, known for the highest levels of quality, integrity, collegiality, and service." It had also defined its core values. To ensure these values were acted upon, the group created a physician compact that codified what the physicians should expect from the group and what the group should expect from the physicians.

DeChant and Mitnick built on the group's prior work on culture and used Lean to achieve the group's vision of national recognition. Many leaders of the group, including its president, were skeptical. They had seen foundation CEOs come and go over the prior decade and felt that the physicians had lost control over care delivery as the successive CEOs focused their attention on controlling the budget and the need to meet system-wide expectations.

Consultant coaches introduced Lean by developing value streams, first in internal medicine and then in the lab, in imaging, and in the call center. Everyone working in these departments, along with the leaders, gradually learned about workflow redesign and A3 thinking and experienced real-life lessons on the challenge of change. Although these departments had achieved a number of improvements, the gains were limited to the departments in which the value streams were located.

Within the first year of the Lean journey, Gould hired a new COO, Katherine Manuel, MAOM, who also saw the potential of Lean transformation. Working together, the CEO, COO, and CMO added the other key components of a Lean management system—Strategy Deployment and the Daily Management System—to spread Lean throughout the organization.

The Strategy Deployment process allowed the group to identify important goals, focus on key metrics, and clarify which leaders were responsible for driving key initiatives. The Daily Management System was created to empower doctors and their support staff to identify and fix problems on the front lines, thus addressing the workflow barriers and frustrations that drive suboptimal performance and burnout.

A major factor in successfully driving the change across the organization was the development of a new management approach that included physician-administrator dyads at multiple levels of the organization. These pairs reported to paired department chairs and managers, who in turn reported to paired divisional medical directors and operations directors. This team reported to the CMO-COO pair, who jointly managed all the clinical services.

Gould invested heavily in training and developing leaders to become mentors and coaches to those they support, to learn how to use visual management and lead huddles effectively, and to design and spread new standard work approaches to workflows. As COO, Manuel now spends half of her time in the *gemba* supporting the teams at the point of care.

It was evident that Gould had undergone a deep and sustained culture change when staff and managers in the department of obstetrics and gynecology launched a new value stream without the support of external consultants. The physicians and staff redesigned and agreed on standard workflows that ensure quality and save considerable time. With the streamlined workflow, the physician now waits in the exam room for the patient to arrive, a real differentiator that drives patient satisfaction.

Gould's improvements have been documented and sustained over time. *Consumer Reports* performs an annual rating of 170 medical groups in California. In 2014 and 2015 Gould received the highest overall rating score in the state. Physician satisfaction improved dramatically as well. In 2011 and 2012, provider satisfaction, based on the AMGA survey, was at the 45th percentile. By 2015 it had climbed steadily to reach the 87th percentile.

Gould, like other physician groups, still faces plenty of challenges, as changes in regulations, payer demands, patient demographics, and technology steadily increase the complexity of the job. Mitnick remains undaunted, though. "We have been wasting the intellectual property of frontline staff for 30 years. A physician's day is enjoyable or not based on staff performance. With the physician and medical assistant working as a team, patients are prepped, the rooms are stocked with everything you need, and the day flows smoothly." As a result, surveyors of the medical group see happy doctors and staff everywhere they go.

*♫*

In this chapter, we've highlighted some organizations that have taken proactive steps to address the problems in the workplace that drive physician burnout. In the next chapter, we'll describe Lean Done Right and explain why we believe it encapsulates all the elements needed for building and maintaining a workplace that energizes physicians rather than burning them out.

## REFERENCES

Friedberg MW, Chen PG, Van Busum KR, et al. Factors affecting physician professional satisfaction and their implications for patient care, health systems, and health policy. RAND Corporation. 2013. Available at: http://www.rand.org/pubs/research_reports/RR439.html. Accessed May 12, 2016.

Gabow PA, Goodman PL. *The Lean Prescription: Powerful Medicine for Our Ailing Healthcare System.* Boca Raton, FL: Productivity Press. 2015:14–18; 136.

Gabow PA, Mehler PS. A broad and structured approach to improving patient safety and quality: lessons from Denver Health. *Health Aff.* 2011;30(4):612–618.

Hafer MS. *Simpler Healthcare: Using Lean to Achieve Breakthrough Improvements in Safety, Quality, Access, and Productivity.* Simpler Healthcare. 2012.

Stanford Hospital and Clinics Medical Staff Update. Worklife and wellness incorporated into practice planning. 2011. Available at: http://med.stanford.edu/shs/update/archives/JULY2011/linzer-speaks.htm. Accessed July 16, 2016.

Walnut Hill Medical Center. About our facility. 2016. Available at: http://www.walnuthillmc.com/about/our-facility.aspx. Accessed July 16, 2016.

# CHAPTER 11
## LEAN DONE RIGHT AS THE WORKPLACE SOLUTION

*Innovation through Lean's proven methods*
*provides hope for better health care at less cost.*
—JOHN S. TOUSSAINT, MD, AND LEONARD
BARRY, PHD, "THE PROMISE OF LEAN IN HEALTH
CARE," *MAYO CLINIC PROCEEDINGS*, 2013

*One thing we didn't realize before we started out was*
*that Lean returns joy to the work, which is something*
*a lot of people in health care don't feel anymore.*
—PATRICIA A. GABOW, MD, FORMER
CEO OF DENVER HEALTH[1]

Leading a Lean transformation is not easy. Many people are suspicious about Lean when they first hear that it's being introduced into their organization. And for good reason. Too often, executives choose to pursue Lean for the wrong reasons and implement Lean in a way that does more harm than good.

Lean can be a positive force, enhancing the personal development and well-being of employees and resulting in dramatic improvements in

---

1 Health Finance Management Association. What Lean can mean to your organization—if it's done right: a conversation with Patricia Gabow, MD. [Blog]. November 2, 2015. Available at: http://www.hfma.org/Leadership/Archives/2015/Fall/What_Lean_Can_Mean_to_Your_Organization%E2%80%94If_It_s_Done_Right. Accessed November 1, 2016.

business performance, or Lean can harm workers in multiple ways and ultimately hurt the organization as well.

In this chapter we'll delve into the key differences between Lean Done Right and, as Mark Graban, Lean consultant and vice president of improvement and innovation services for the software company KaiNexus, has called it, Lean As Misguidedly Executed, or "L.A.M.E."

## BACKGROUND

Lean has improved the performance of organizations within manufacturing, the service industry, the military, and health care. James P. Womack and Daniel T. Jones succinctly described the benefits of Lean in a 1994 *Harvard Business Review* article. "By eliminating unnecessary steps, aligning all steps in an activity in a continuous flow, recombining labor into cross-functional teams dedicated to that activity, and continually striving for improvement, companies can develop, produce, and distribute products with *half or less* of the human effort, space, tools, time, and overall expense. They can also become vastly more flexible and responsive to customer desires." (Womack 1994)

Manufacturing companies that adopt Lean effectively are more competitive, experiencing a 10 to 12 percent increase in revenue and a 12 to 15 percent increase in income, according to one author. (Ransom 2008) Another study found that organizations that implement Lean comprehensively are three times more likely to achieve a best-in-industry distinction. (Bartels 2005)

And yet the majority of organizations that implement Lean fail to reach their targeted goals.

A Wall Street analyst famously stated that only 1 to 2 percent of companies that implement Lean do so effectively enough to experience financial benefits. (Hall; no date) Others have documented *negative* effects from introducing Lean, including increased worker stress and reduced job satisfaction. (Parker 2001)

What is the explanation for the disconnect between the organizations that see benefits across a wide range of performance metrics and those that fail to see benefits or that experience negative effects? We believe the key distinctions are the degree to which Lean is embraced by leaders and the degree to which the organization implements Lean as it was originally intended, which is deeply based in the two Lean principles of Respect for People and Continuous Improvement. We view Respect for People to be the more important of the two principles, because you can achieve *improvement* without Respect for People, but it's not likely to be *continuous* unless there is deeply rooted respect for workers. We refer to this approach as "Lean Done Right."

Lean experts agree. To quote John Toussaint and Leonard Berry in a 2013 article: "Lean is not a program; it is not a set of quality improvement tools; it is not a quick fix; it is not a responsibility that can be delegated. Rather, Lean is a cultural transformation that changes how an organization works." (Toussaint 2013)

Kimberly Petty is CEO of Zoetify and co-founder of Vocera's Experience Innovation Network, which is a community to support the adoption of innovations to improve the human connection in health care. She told us,

> What we have witnessed in many organizations is "Lean" focused on cost reduction that is demoralizing and emotionally draining to the staff—contributing to burnout. However, I intentionally put Lean in quotes, because what is usually going on in these organizations is that individuals are utilizing some of the Lean process improvement tools but failing to deploy the Lean management system and a culture of employee empowerment that enables the removal of barriers and frustration. I am a Lean Six Sigma Master Black Belt who absolutely believes in Lean, but only Lean done right and Lean that not only strips out waste but that also seeks to put something back in to address the gaps in compassion, communication, emotional support, and humanity that are essential to providing high quality care.

Petty's mentor, Bridget Duffy, MD, chief medical officer at Vocera and co-founder of The Experience Innovation Network, said in an interview, "The 'leanification' and 'appification' of health care is not solving for the root cause of burnout among physicians and nurses. Lean is transformative only when it removes waste and then hardwires in something positive in its place, like empathy. Being told, 'Work harder, work smarter, work faster with less money, and now look up and smile at the patient,' breeds cynicism."

## WHAT LEAN IS *NOT*

We have learned through our interviews and Paul's coaching work that many physicians and administrators have negative impressions of Lean, from either direct experience or word of mouth. What we have come to recognize is the degree to which Lean is misunderstood. Given the misunderstandings about Lean and the prevalence of negative connotations of Lean, it's important that we begin by addressing some of these objections and misconceptions.

*Objection #1: Patients are not cars. Lean won't work in health care.* It's true that Lean was developed for improving performance in automobile manufacturing (more on that later). However, health care does share some characteristics with other fields in which Lean has been successfully applied, namely, aviation and nuclear energy. All three are complex fields in which errors can have life-threatening consequences. Lean, when implemented as a comprehensive system, has been highly effective in health care.

*Objection #2: Lean is about standardizing. I don't want to practice cookbook medicine.* Physicians value autonomy for good reasons. There are many times when a physician must use his or her best judgment to independently decide and act on what is right for the patient. As we have described earlier, physicians undergo decades of training and continuous learning to be prepared to make and carry out such decisions when necessary.

Standard Work is a key component of process improvement in Lean. Many physicians fear that standardization will reduce their autonomy, equating it with the term *practice guidelines* that emerged in the 1990s as a way to address the high degree of practice variation among physicians in the treatment of patients with the same diagnosis. Initially, physicians felt the guidelines were a direct threat to the autonomy required to address the unique needs of each patient. However, over time, they saw that implementing standards of practice in a way that recognizes both the uniqueness of each patient and the commonalities between patients is in the best interest of the patient.

In Lean, Standard Work is defined as:

> *The currently best-known way to perform a specific task, designed by the people who do the work, with the expectation that the workers will continuously improve the standard over time.*

Understood this way, Standard Work actually empowers workers by encouraging them not to simply accept the standard process as written but to improve the standard process using Lean process improvement tools such as RIEs and A3s, which we'll explain later in this chapter. Thus, Standard Work is not static but continuously evolving as conditions change or as workers gain more experience and better understanding of the problem.

*Misconception #1: Lean is a set of performance improvement tools focused solely on efficiency.* Quite often, administrators and clinicians think of Lean as being a specific improvement tool or set of tools. When used this way, it is rarely sustainable. In fact, when Lean is applied as an improvement tool alone, it may *worsen* burnout if the clinical team becomes overwhelmed or demoralized when being held accountable for performance metrics related to "Lean" projects without sufficient resources to improve those metrics. Lean is more than a few performance improvement tools. It is a philosophy, an approach, an effective mechanism for culture change, a leadership and management system, and a means for whole enterprise transformation.

As Toussaint and his co-authors stated in a 2016 Health Affairs article, much confusion exists regarding Lean and its true components. (Toussaint 2016)

> It is true that what has been called the Toyota Production System in the past may have failed at some health care institutions. Therein lies the problem. National standards for applying TPS in health care have not been established. However, the sheer number of organizations and physicians that are seeking

to understand this methodology suggests it has real merit. The fact that some organizations as noted are reporting excellent results is the attraction...Early evidence is encouraging but there is more work to do.

Lean Done Right is a comprehensive system and approach that transforms an organization into a collective of problem-solvers. Workers are empowered to identify and remove the barriers and frustrations in their workplace and are engaged to do meaningful work. Lean Done Right is about leaders listening to and empowering workers as much as it is about specific improvement tools.

*Misconception #2: Lean leads to layoffs and fewer resources to do our jobs.* "Lean is mean" is a belief based on the too-often-realized fear that becoming more efficient equates to loss of jobs. We believe that when this happens, it reflects an incomplete adoption of Lean, usually based on a lack of understanding of what Lean, as fully conceived, entails. Removing barriers and frustrations in the workplace is not "mean," and Lean does not need to result in a reduction in personnel. In fact, Lean experts recommend that organizations implement a no-layoff policy before starting a Lean journey.

As Womack stated in an online forum in response to criticism that Lean results in the elimination of jobs, "As I look at the world, we have an enormous surplus of *muda* (waste) in every industry and human activity. At the same time, we have an enormous shortage of resources to deal with issues ranging from global security and climate change, to AIDS and living standards in the developing countries, to health care for aging populations in the developed countries. Our challenge is to convert the waste required to perform many current activities into new capacity to perform needed activities. So Lean thinking must be a big part of the solution. By itself, Lean can't be mean." (Womack 2003)

In our interview, Womack emphasized his concern about misconceptions of Lean. "We don't want a lay notion of Lean—'work harder'— to be confused with Lean. People sometimes refer to Lean as mean or green. But beyond the word is confusion about Lean being about 'the screws being put on.'" Harvard Business School professor David Upton has said, "Some people think Lean means 'not fat,' as in laying people off." He and colleagues argue that instead Lean changes how a company learns through new ways to solve problems, coordinate activities, and standardize processes. (Hanna 2007)

Creating the Lean organizational culture and incorporating the Lean philosophy of Respect for People are absolutely essential to Lean Done Right. Given the importance of understanding what Lean Done Right entails, we'll describe the philosophy and key principles of Lean.

## LEAN PHILOSOPHY

Toyota originally created TPS to design and build cars. TPS evolved not through a pre-thought master plan but through experimentation and trial and error, which ultimately shaped Toyota's structure and management system. (Shimokawa 2009) Both TPS and Lean share a core philosophy that focuses on maximizing value from the customer's perspective by identifying and removing waste. As Toussaint and Berry wrote in an article in *Mayo Clinic Proceedings*, "The underlying goal of Lean in health care is to improve value for patients. Doing so should also benefit other health care stakeholders. Fewer medication errors, fewer nosocomial infections, less nursing time away from the bedside, faster operating room turnover time, improved care team communication about patients, and faster response time for emergent cases not only [benefits] patients but also physicians, nurses, health care organizations, payers, and the community." (Toussaint 2013)

A core element of the Lean philosophy is valuing and investing in workers. A primary goal of Lean is building the capacity of workers to identify and design effective solutions for problems in their daily work environment.

Lean experts have identified eight sources of waste, which can be recalled with the mnemonic TRIMWOOD. The following list names these sources along with common examples in health care:

- **T**ransport—Moving patients from room to room in an office or unit
- **H**uman **R**esources—Unused human potential, as when physicians enter data into the EHR

- Inventory—Secret stashes of supplies kept in a local environment due to fear of running out and delays in restocking
- Movement (unnecessary)—Needing to leave a room to get commonly used supplies or equipment
- Waiting—A full waiting room; frequent delays in surgery start times
- Overproduction—Repeating tests because results are not available
- Overprocessing—Repeatedly filling out or signing forms
- Defects—Prescribing errors, wound infections, inaccurate progress notes

## PRINCIPLES OF LEAN

Lean is a management system and philosophy based on two simple principles: Continuous Improvement and Respect for People. In this section, we'll describe these principles. Too often, leaders and managers focus on the former to the exclusion of the latter. Both are necessary for sustained improvement—and for preventing physician burnout. We'll also describe Lean leadership and a Lean management system, two essential aspects of Lean Done Right.

### Continuous Improvement

The philosophy of Continuous Improvement has characterized Lean since its inception as TPS. A primary goal of Lean is creating a mind-set and capacity in every worker such that continually looking for places to improve is second nature. Workers are empowered to use a scientific method to complete small tests of change in their daily work. They come to see their work responsibilities as two-fold: doing the work and improving on the work.

The principle of continuously improving the service or product provided to a customer is vital to an organization's long-term survival and success. Continuous Improvement is also empowering to workers, because they improve both outcomes and their work environment by removing waste, decreasing chaos, and improving teamwork.

## Respect for People

Respect for People is a vital Lean principle that is commonly overlooked. Too often, health care leaders rush to implement the Continuous Improvement principle of Lean with practices and tools to identify and fix waste, but they forget Respect for People and thus ultimately undermine the long-term success of Lean at their organizations.

As Richard Zarbo, MD, DMD, senior vice president and chair of pathology and laboratory medicine at Henry Ford Health System, wrote in an editorial, "Most imitators of Lean use a top-down directed approach to projects by using selected improvement and work design tools often wielded by quality professionals or consultants. I believe this misses the critical element of Toyota's success, namely creating a workplace culture that is educated, engaged, trusted, structured, and incentivized to participate." (Zarbo 2012)

The principle of Respect for People stems from an idea inherent in the original design of the Toyota manufacturing process and expressed by Fujio Cho, its former chairman, "First we build people, then we build cars." (Keller 2008) Toyota believed strongly in investing in its employees. At its core, this philosophy necessitates a culture change that engages those who do the work in continuous problem-solving.

When acting in concert with this principle, leaders take a different stance with workers. They invest in enabling and empowering frontline workers to be problem-solvers. They manage by coaching, not disciplining. They ensure that they understand the daily experience of the frontline worker and prioritize the improvement of that experience. They institute a no-layoff policy with any performance improvement initiative. And they see *systems*, not *people*, as the source of problems in the organization.

Respect for People also includes creating an organization that supports healthy work-life balance. Leaders acting on this principle don't just pay lip service to valuing workers but actually treat them as important assets. Holding the value of Respect for People is foundational for creating a healthy organization, which decreases the risk of physician burnout. As Monica Broome at the University of Miami told us, "Ensuring a culture of respect is not a huge drain on finances or work-intense. It is a high-impact, low-investment 'intervention' that makes a huge difference."

The principle of Respect for People is foundational to success with Lean. Organizations can achieve improvement with many different Lean approaches, but without a focus on the principle of Respect for People, achievements are unlikely to be sustained.

Leaders fail to demonstrate Respect for People when they:

- Use layoffs to improve financial performance (and perhaps fail to recognize that layoffs never improve quality or service)
- Instruct frontline workers to implement best practices without providing them with needed resources or acknowledging the barriers to implementation
- Do not spend time with frontline workers to truly understand the challenges of doing the work
- Make the manager's role difficult by insisting that he or she motivate frontline workers and deliver stellar results without providing needed support and resources

Many of the Lean experts we interviewed emphasized the importance of Respect for People in an organization's ultimate success in achieving the benefits of Lean. Kimberly Petty at Zoetify told us, "When I arrived at Cleveland Clinic from General Electric as a Lean Six Sigma black belt, I realized that using Lean to strip out waste wasn't going to do it. You have to have human factors involved. They are going to define the outcome. Nowhere is this more true than in health care."

Bob Chapman at Barry-Wehmiller told us he dislikes the name "Lean" because it doesn't acknowledge the core philosophy of valuing employees. "It should be called 'Listen.' Its power is to listen to people and validate their worth, to listen and ask them how to do the work better." He went on to say that his leadership strategy places respect for workers as a top priority. As he put it, "My priorities are people, then purpose, then performance. This is not the case in most workplaces. This applies everywhere, including health care and the military. I care about the care we give in a hospital *and* about the caregivers. They are just as important as the patient."

Gene Lindsey, formerly at Atrius Health, identified the principle of Respect for People as a unique strength of Lean. He said, "Only in a collective effort like Lean can you actually come together and create a system that respects people, and where their ideas are incorporated and has as a goal of efficiency that includes mission."

In her book *The Lean Prescription: Powerful Medicine for Our Ailing Healthcare System,* Patricia Gabow, formerly at Denver Health, describes the connection between Lean's focus on removal of waste and the principle of Respect for People. She and her co-author write that waste is disrespectful: (Gabow 2015)

- To humanity because it squanders scarce resources
- To workers because it asks them to do work with no value
- To patients because it asks them to endure processes of no value
- To citizens because it asks them to pay taxes for work with no value

Without effective leadership neither Continuous Improvement nor Respect for People will gain true traction within an organization. Leaders must have a deep understanding of Lean and fully engage in Lean principles and components for Lean to make any headway. In an interview, Chapman emphasized that caring about workers is also a sound business strategy. "It's not about nice. It's about creating the sense that workers feel safe and valued, that what they do matters. In business school, we are taught to follow numbers, not how to show we care. What we've demonstrated is that you can care about people *and* create value for all stakeholders and thrive as an organization. It is a rich balance between a good business model and a caring culture."

Next, we'll discuss a critical element for successful adoption of Lean: leadership.

## LEAN LEADERSHIP
The successful adoption of Lean and the achievement of improved performance metrics hinge on an organization's leadership. We've seen that when executives fail to fully engage in Lean themselves, the result is mediocre at best. At worst, the result can cause more harm than good. If administration uses a top-down management approach to implement

Lean and dictates that performance metrics will be achieved (and rewards or penalties exacted) without the input and engagement of frontline clinicians, this violates the principle of Respect for People and is unlikely to result in long-term success.

Lean will often be introduced into an organization in a single department by a motivated manager. If managers or clinical teams attempt to use Lean tools in isolation and without the full engagement of other departments and service lines, they will not realize the full potential of Lean and may risk losing their jobs if their Lean approach to management is out of sync with the organization's leadership.

Lindsey described the importance of Lean Leadership in an online article posted in 2016: (Lindsey 2016)

Lean is misunderstood if it is just used as a collection of tools to solve urgent problems over the next few financial cycles. No doubt Lean can create sustainable competency with breakthrough accomplishments. Despite what Lean can accomplish, an organization is wasting money if the CEO and senior management can offer no more than casual support or are just tolerant of Lean. Worse yet is when the CEO tries to tap into the benefits of Lean by proxy through others while continuing the traditional "Sloan Management" top-down process of management by objective. If the reality is that the CEO and senior leaders do not effectively do the standard work of Lean leadership, it would be better for the organization to buy lottery tickets than spend money and effort trying to implement Lean with leadership sitting on the side lines.

For Lean to be effective, leaders must take an active role. They must undertake a personal transformation and eschew a top-down leadership style. They must fully understand and engage in Lean. They must prioritize Lean transformation and direct needed resources toward Lean initiatives. Lean leadership changes an organization's culture. As shown in figure 3, Lean culture differs in many aspects from traditional culture.

Lean culture embodies many elements that address the workplace problems that are the underlying root causes of physician burnout. Leadership style is critical to successful adoption of Lean.

| Traditional Culture | Lean Culture |
|---|---|
| Function Silos | Interdisciplinary teams |
| Managers direct | Managers teach/enable |
| Benchmark to justify not improving: "just as good" | Seek the ultimate performance, the absence of waste |
| Blame people | Root cause analysis |
| Rewards: individual | Rewards: group sharing |
| Supplier is enemy | Supplier is ally |
| Guard information | Share information |
| Volume lowers cost | Removing waste lowers cost |
| Internal focus | Customer focus |
| Expert driven | Process driven |

Figure 3. Traditional Culture versus Lean Culture

Table used with permission from Arthur P. Byrne and Orest Fiume.

Lean leadership style is based on the concepts of servant leadership and full engagement of leaders. Servant leadership is the polar opposite of the top-down, traditional management style. Servant leadership focuses on supporting and enabling the individuals whose work adds value to the customer—in this case, the patient and his or her family. As James Hereford of Stanford University Medical Center put it, "Success requires leaders who empower workers to make changes and provide help with direction on where to focus."

Lean leadership style also requires full engagement in Lean. As Lindsey put it, "The leader cannot be above or outside the Lean process and expect it to work. People pay far more attention to what they see you doing than what they hear you saying." In a similar vein, Graban wrote, "Impressive and sustainable Lean results come from organizations where the CEO and leaders at all levels embrace Lean as a way of managing and a way of guiding daily decisions and improvement activities." (Graban 2012)

Perhaps Lean Leadership is best summed up by the famous quote attributed to Mahatma Gandhi: "Be the change you wish to see in the world."

## LEAN MANAGEMENT SYSTEM

In this section, we'll present a brief summary of a Lean management system (LMS) and its components. For a more in-depth description of LMS, please review the recommended reading list in Appendix 1.

A Lean management system is often viewed as having four key components:

- Strategy Deployment
- Value Stream Improvement
- Daily Management System
- Lean support infrastructure

All four components are critical to a successful Lean transformation. We'll provide an overview of each component. In the next chapter, we'll show how Lean organizations use these components as part of an integrated management system.


## Strategy Deployment

Strategy Deployment (SD) is the process by which a Lean organization sets its strategy and ensures that the tactics necessary to achieve the strategic goals are defined and achieved.

To begin SD, the leadership team defines the organization's long-term (three- to five-year) goals and the metrics by which progress toward these goals will be measured. Most Lean organizations refer to these as True North Metrics, or TNMs. Leaders create specific metrics, based directly on the organization's TNMs, for each level of the enterprise. These measures are referred to as tiered TNMs.

The leadership team then assigns goals and tactics to the appropriate departments and units of the organization and, through an iterative process, determines metrics for each goal. The process ensures that each department, unit, and team in the organization has specific and clearly understandable goals and has the capability to deliver on those goals.


## Value Stream Improvement

The value stream is a set of activities that an organization performs to deliver a product or service. In health care, the value stream is all the tasks performed by workers in the health care organization to provide health care services to patients. Value Stream Improvement (VSI) is the activity that many people with limited exposure to Lean Done Right consider to be synonymous with Lean. In VSI, a team composed mostly of people who work in the value stream analyze every step from start to finish, identifying and removing any waste or defects.

The bulk of this work is done in week-long *Kaizen* or Rapid Improvement Events (RIEs). RIEs bring together a team with expertise in the workflow in the *gemba* (or "the place where work is done") and expertise in key support areas, such as IT and finance. The team follows an A3 problem-solving process to understand the root causes of the problem and implement changes to address them. (See Appendix 2 for an illustration of this process.) The A3 process includes steps for follow-up to ensure full implementation of the solution and to assess its effectiveness in addressing the identified problem.

## Daily Management System

The Daily Management System (DMS) is a set of processes used by leaders, managers, and frontline workers to support the effectiveness and stability of operations across the organization. The DMS consists of daily huddles in each local unit that ensure the unit is ready for the day, is on track to achieve its performance targets as aligned with the TNMs, and is able to solve local problems that frontline workers have identified. Problems that cannot be solved locally are escalated to the next level in the organization through tiered huddles. Tiered huddles are daily gatherings that occur at each level of the organization—generally three to five tiers. These huddles provide a structure in which information can flow from the front lines to the C-suite and from the top leaders to frontline clinicians. Problems that cannot be solved locally are escalated, even up to the CEO if necessary, to ensure that adequate attention and resources are provided to solve them.

## Lean support infrastructure

The Lean support infrastructure includes personnel who enable the work of Lean coaches, who, in turn, provide education about Lean and support Lean activities across the organization. It also includes personnel in various departments whose expertise is key to successful Lean transformation, such as:

- Human resources—to develop leadership and support the redeployment employees into new roles as processes become more efficient, and their original positions are made redundant
- Decision support—to provide timely and specific metrics to each unit and level in the organization
- Finance—to ensure the organization is achieving the projected financial targets necessary to keep the business viable

The leadership team of the organization is responsible for ensuring that all four components of the Lean management system are well coordinated and functioning effectively.

## THE POWER OF LEAN DONE RIGHT

Lean Done Right brings together a leadership approach, a culture change, and a variety of tools that create a nimble, efficient organization—one that is also a healthy workplace for everyone, including physicians. In this section, we'll describe the power of Lean Done Right to fix what's broken in health care and address the workplace drivers of physician burnout.

Lean Done Right empowers leaders and workers to create a healthy workplace. It builds the practice environment and organizational culture and structure that neutralize the workplace drivers of burnout. As a reminder, the comprehensive list of workplace drivers (described in Chapters 4 through 7) of burnout for physicians include:

- Work overload
- Lack of control
- Insufficient reward
- Breakdown of community
- Absence of fairness
- Conflicting values
- Chaos and inefficiencies

- Undue clerical burden
- Time pressure
- Work-life imbalance
- Loss of meaning in work
- Top-down leadership
- EHR

## Lean Done Right creates a healthy organizational culture through Lean leadership

As we discussed in Chapter 6, leaders have a significant impact on the workplace drivers of burnout. By fully embracing the principle of Respect for People, Lean leaders set the stage for creating a healthy organizational culture. Lean leadership, with its emphasis on coaching rather than employing a top-down, control-and-command style, generates a positive environment that directly influences the environment at the front lines of care.

The creation of a healthy organizational culture impacts several workplace drivers of burnout, as shown below:

- Insufficient reward
- Breakdown of community
- Absence of fairness
- Conflicting values
- Top-down leadership

## Lean Done Right empowers and engages workers

Lean Done Right empowers and engages workers in several ways. Standard Work is developed by the people who do the work. When Standard Work is implemented, the frontline clinicians identify any unanticipated consequences of the new Standard Work, and they test solutions to continuously improve it. RIEs involve workers and leaders at all levels. As Gabow said in an online interview, "I'm not a 'touchy-feely' sort of person, but the first time I saw a clerk stand up proudly to address a big group of people, including leadership, at a report-out from an RIE, it almost brought tears to my eyes." (Phillips 2014) The use of strategy deployment in the form of tiered TNMs and tiered huddles creates an organization in which everyone is pulling in the same direction and a dependable channel exists for communication between leadership and the front lines.

Gabow described the connection between Lean and empowerment in *The Lean Prescription*: "In my 40 years in health care, Lean is the only approach I have seen that truly empowers everyone and converts empowerment from a meaningless catchphrase to an operational reality." (Gabow 2015)

Participation in Lean events and problem-solving on the front lines provide opportunities for personal improvement, which engenders a sense of control. David Fillingham, former chief executive at the Royal Bolton Hospital in the United Kingdom, told us of the connection he sees between involving workers in improvement efforts and the prevention of burnout. "Lack of control and overburden contribute to burnout. Engaging staff to improve the quality of care can help with burnout."

In our interview, Graban described the importance of investing the time to fully involve workers in improving their work. "Principle number one of the Toyota Way is to do things for the long term; in the short term, it might be more time-consuming and expensive to get everyone to hash through it, but Toyota has found that the people doing the work need to write the Standard Work. I don't think they said that because it was benevolent, but because their experience has shown it's effective." He continued by pointing out the practical implications of such an approach, saying, "When people get to participate in standard work discussions, the improvement process goes more smoothly."

Research suggests that empowering physicians in the clinical setting can help reduce burnout. Mark Linzer at Hennepin County Medical Center and his colleagues conducted a randomized study of 34 primary care clinics. (Linzer 2015) Clinicians in the study group met with the researchers to choose the interventions they wanted to pursue. When resurveyed 12 to 18 months after implementing the chosen interventions, more physicians in the study clinics showed a decrease in burnout and an increase in satisfaction than physicians in the control clinics. The research team identified two categories of interventions that were more likely to be associated with reductions in physician burnout: workflow redesign and implementing improvement projects targeting quality metrics, medication reconciliation, and screening processes.

Empowering and engaging workers has a direct impact on the following drivers of burnout:

- Lack of control
- Breakdown of community
- Loss of meaning in work

## Lean Done Right removes wasteful activities and inefficiencies at the front lines

Lean Done Right removes waste from workflow processes, which allows workers to get more done in less time with fewer resources and fewer defects. A commonly used adage in Lean transformation is "double the good and halve the bad." In some cases, a redesign reduces the time required for a process or task by less than 50 percent, but in other cases teams cut the required time by 75 to 90 percent.

By reducing the time required to complete each task, the overall workload decreases as well. For physicians, the reduction in time per task translates into greater ease in getting through their schedule and completing the work day. As Fillingham put it, "Lean's specific focus on waste leads to better outcomes for patient and easier work for staff." Given that many physicians now work two to four hours each evening to complete chart notes, refill requests, and referral authorizations, the first effect for physicians of process redesign through Lean Done Right is likely to be a reduction in their "after-hours" work and in the time they spend away from family.

For this reason, removing wasteful activities and inefficiencies in the practice environment has a major impact on improving work-life balance for clinicians. After a Lean transformation at Northeast Georgia Medical Group, which we mentioned in Chapter 10, James Murphey, the internist and pediatrician, found previously "lost" time. During an RIE, the team rearranged the daily schedule to account for triage and documentation time. Murphey said, "Before the change, I was happy if

I managed to be just 30 to 45 minutes behind in my schedule and was taking home two to three hours of work for the evenings. Now, if I'm 10 to 15 minutes behind, I feel I might do better. I don't feel as guilty for keeping my patients waiting. At home I might have 15 to 30 minutes of work to do, and many days I have none."

As the time required for tasks decreases, physicians are better able to stay on time with their schedule, reducing the pressure they feel from falling behind. As Murphey described it, "The new process with Lean keeps us on time with patients with routine illnesses and conditions, so we have more time for patients with complex conditions." Improving physicians' ability to stay on time benefits them and their patients. Physicians feel less pressure and guilt about making their patients wait. Patients experience less wasted time and are less likely to feel that physicians are hurrying or short-changing them during their visit.

Removing waste and inefficiencies at the front lines directly addresses the following key workplace drivers of burnout:

- Work overload
- Chaos and inefficiencies
- Undue clerical burden
- EHR
- Time pressure
- Work-life imbalance
- Loss of meaning in work

**Lean Done Right cuts across silos to fix enterprise-wide problems**
Lean Done Right helps organizations and individual teams identify the root causes of waste in their daily processes. Often the discovery work leads teams to cross operational silos to address the root causes.

As an example, in many organizations, defects in the process of managing appointment scheduling and messaging often frustrate workers in both the call center and clinical care centers. Pulling together a team that consists of leaders and frontline workers from both entities to work on a problem-solving A3 could fix the problem in a way that fosters the discovery of unique, effective solutions that neither entity would have identified on its own.

Tiered huddles and strategy deployment are other ways that Lean Done Right fosters organization-wide communication and collaboration toward similar goals.

Lindsey described his first experience with an RIE as eye opening for him about this aspect of Lean. He said, "Our first event was focused on the inpatient admissions process. We began to see waste and to fix some of the problems that physicians were dealing with over and over again. Gradually, I became aware of the ability of Lean to cut across the silos in our organization. I also saw that while rudimentary Lean, meaning just the Lean tools, can improve a great deal within a silo, it can't cut across silos the way a comprehensive Lean transformation can."

By cutting across silos to fix enterprise-wide problems, Lean Done Right addresses the following workplace drivers of burnout:

- Breakdown of community
- Absence of fairness
- Chaos and inefficiencies

## Lean Done Right creates a highly adaptable organization

Lean transformation creates an organization that can rapidly adapt to external changes. An organization with the capacity to more quickly adapt will be less likely to be one in which physicians are roiled by the waves of external factors that put pressure on the health care organization and increase the risk of burnout. This capacity confers a distinct advantage especially in competitive markets.

In response to a change in regulations or market dynamics, fully developed Lean organizations can choose a new strategy and implement it quickly. As Leon C. Megginson, a professor of business at Louisiana State University, famously summarized Charles Darwin's work, "It is not the strongest of the species that survive, nor the most intelligent, but the one most responsive to change." (Quote Investigator 2014) Knowing your organization is likely to respond effectively (and more effectively than its competitors) to external forces can be quite reassuring to leaders and to clinicians.

The creation of a highly adaptable organization helps to address the external factors that put pressure on organizations and affects several workplace drivers of burnout, including the following:

- Work overload
- Lack of control
- Insufficient reward
- Undue clerical burden
- EHR
- Time pressure
- Work-life imbalance

## A CAVEAT

Lean Done Right is not a quick fix. It is not an efficiency tool to reach a short-term target at the expense of balanced improvement. It is a long-term commitment to organizational transformation. Lean must be implemented with care. Using a few specific Lean tools without Lean leadership, the principle of Respect for People, and a Lean management system can do more harm than good. Such an approach could very well increase clinician burnout by heaping additional, poorly conceived improvement projects on health care providers who are doomed to fail because of the flaws in the underlying processes. Dike Drummond, the physician coach and author, has witnessed this scenario in his consulting work. "I've seen Lean blow up. Just half implemented and then there's a mutiny." James Hereford of Stanford University Medical Center concurs. He told us that "Bad Lean, meaning poorly understood Lean, can do great damage, and there is way too much of that being perpetrated."

The engagement of leaders in transformation, including the transformation of their own leadership style, is critical here. In fact, the ThedaCare Center for Healthcare Value, which supports organizations in Lean transformation as exemplified by ThedaCare, no longer provides support to organizations whose senior leaders are not fully engaged in Lean. Toussaint told us that he and his colleagues have found that without such engagement, the investments in money, time, and human capital are just not fruitful.

∭

We firmly believe that Lean Done Right holds tremendous promise for creating not only work environments in which physicians and their co-workers can thrive but also fiscally sound organizations that provide high-quality care and are resilient to the many waves of change in the current health care arena. In the next chapter, we'll recommend specific action steps that organizational leaders, their boards of directors, and individual physicians can take to address the workplace drivers of burnout. We'll also provide physicians with tips to take an active role in improving their relationships with administration to instigate change in their organizations.

## REFERENCES

Bartels, N. Lean in the most generic sense. *Manufact Bus Technol* 2005;23:32–36.

Gabow PA, Goodman PL. *The Lean Prescription: Powerful Medicine for Our Ailing Healthcare System.* Boca Raton, FL: Productivity Press. 2015:14–18.

Graban M. Be Lean, not L.A.M.E. In: Grunden N, Hagood C, eds. *Lean-Led Hospital Design: Creating the Efficient Hospital of the Future.* Boca Raton, FL: Productivity Press. 2012:265–269.

Hall R. Lean manufacturing—fat cash flow: an interview with Clifford F. Ransom II. [Internet]. Available at: http://www.maskell.com/lean_accounting/industry/fat_cash_flow.html. Accessed July 18, 2016.

Hanna J. Bringing "Lean" principles to service industries. Harvard Business School. [Internet]. 2007. Available at: http://hbswk.hbs.edu/item/bringing-lean-principles-to-service-industries. Accessed July 20, 2016.

Keller R. Continuous improvement—what ever happened to respect for people? A successful Lean transformation requires a commitment to the people who make it possible. [Internet]. 2008.

Available at: http://www.industryweek.com/public-policy/contin-uous-improvement-what-ever-happened-respect-people. Accessed July 18, 2016.

Lindsey G. Dr. Gene Lindsey's Healthcare Musings Newsletter. [Internet]. March 18, 2016. Available at: http://strategyhealthcare.com/cat-egory/healthcare-musings-archive. Accessed September 8, 2016.

Linzer M, Poplau S, Grossman E, et al. A cluster randomized trial of interventions to improve work conditions and clinician burnout in primary care: results from the Healthy Work Place (HWP) study. *J Gen Intern Med.* 2015;30(8):1105–1111

Parker S. Longitudinal effects of Lean production on employee out-comes and the mediating role of work characteristics. *J Appl Psychol.* 2001;88(4):620–634.

Phillips L. What Lean can mean to your organization—if it's done right: a conversation with Patricia Gabow, MD. [Internet]. November 2, 2015. Available at: http://www.hfma.org/Leadership/Archives/2015/Fall/What_Lean_Can_Mean_to_Your_Organization%E2%80%94If_It_s_Done_Right/. Accessed July 12, 2016.

Quote Investigator. It is not the strongest of the species that survives but the most adaptable. [Internet]. 2014. Available at: http://quotein-vestigator.com/2014/05/04/adapt/. Accessed July 18, 2016.

Ransom, C. Lean Enterprise Institute. Wall Street view of lean transfor-mation. 2008. Available at: http://www.Lean.org/events. Accessed April 14, 2014.

Shimokawa K, Fujimoto T, eds. *The Birth of Lean.* Cambridge, MA: Lean Enterprise Institute. 2009.

Toussaint J, Conway PH, Shortell SM. The Toyota Production System: what does it mean, and what does it mean for health care? Health Affairs blog. [Internet]. 2016. Available at: http://healthaffairs.org/blog/2016/04/06/the-toyota-production-system-what-does-it-mean-and-what-does-it-mean-for-health-care/. Accessed July 20, 2016.

Toussaint JS, Berry LL. The promise of Lean in health care. *Mayo Clin Proc.* 2013;88(1):74–82.

Womack JP. Is Lean mean? [Internet]. 2003. Available at: http://www.lean.org/womack/DisplayObject.cfm?o=715. Accessed July 18, 2016.

Womack JP, Jones DT. From Lean production to the Lean enterprise. *Harvard Business Review.* March–April 1994. Available at: https://hbr.org/1994/03/from-lean-production-to-the-lean-enterprise. Accessed July 18, 2016.

Zarbo R. Creating and sustaining a lean culture of continuous process improvement. *Am J Clin Pathol.* 2012;138:321–326.

# CHAPTER 12

## ACTION PLANS FOR LEADERS, BOARDS, AND PHYSICIANS

*Every system is perfectly designed to get the results it gets.*
—PAUL B. BATALDEN, MD, SENIOR FELLOW,
INSTITUTE FOR HEALTHCARE IMPROVEMENT[1]

*The principles of team-based performance improvement
and participatory management have a role in
preventing burnout and improving engagement.*
—STEPHEN J. SWENSEN, MD, MEDICAL DIRECTOR FOR
LEADERSHIP AND ORGANIZATION DEVELOPMENT AT MAYO CLINIC

Burnout threatens the sustainability of our health care delivery system, the well-being and engagement of health care professionals, and the quality and safety of the care that patients receive. If the hospital or medical group that you lead or in which you practice is typical, more than half of physicians are experiencing burnout symptoms, and the vast majority of physicians and staff think that their leaders don't care.

The most effective way to prevent physician burnout is to change the organizational structure and processes that lead to burnout—those drivers that we described in Chapters 3 through 8. However, most health

---

1 Like Magic? Institute for Healthcare Improvement. Available at: http://www.ihi.org/
communities/blogs/_layouts/ihi/community/blog/itemview.aspx?List=7d1126ec-8f63-
4a3b-9926-c44ea3036813&ID=159. Accessed September 22, 2016.

care leaders are concerned that the changes typically recommended to reduce the risk of physician burnout—for example, decreasing the number of patients seen per day, taking more time off, or participating in wellness activities—will also reduce revenues or increase expenses, putting the financial viability of the organization at risk. The irony is that *not* addressing physician burnout is a recipe for putting the organization's fiscal health in jeopardy, for the reasons we described in Chapter 2.

We wish we could tell you that there is a single, easy solution to the problem of physician burnout, but that is not the case. Physician burnout is driven by a multitude of underlying root causes for which there are no quick fixes. A health care organization that leaps into strategies to address burnout without fully understanding the root causes in each clinical setting is unlikely to successfully create a healthy workplace that is adaptable to external pressures and can prevent burnout over the long term.

For this reason, we are *not* presenting a generic checklist of best practices or innovative ideas for addressing burnout. Instead, we present our recommendations for beginning a journey to understand and address the drivers of burnout in each individual setting. We strongly believe that Lean Done Right effectively addresses both the drivers of physician burnout and the underlying problems that prevent organizations from achieving the Triple Aim. Lean Done Right allows each organization to foster an environment in which leaders, managers, and frontline clinicians can work in partnership to address the workplace drivers of burnout.

The target state is one in which the workplace is efficient, stable, and reliable; where people treat each other with respect, where frontline clinicians and managers solve problems rapidly, where all stakeholders are aligned around caring for the patient and striving to achieve optimal quality, cost, and service, and where physicians are engaged in all aspects of work redesign and continuous improvement. We have seen the transformative effects of creating such work environments.

## A CALL TO ACTION: LEADERS FIRST

Executive leaders need to take action to address burnout, but not with the traditional management approach that has created the problem.

We propose that the leadership approach embodied in Lean Done Right will prevent physician burnout while significantly improving the organization's performance and its short- and long-term viability. As we described in previous chapters, it is a leadership approach built upon the two key principles of Lean: Respect for People and Continuous Improvement.

These two key principles of Lean Done Right are exemplified by the actions taken by the organizations described in Chapter 10 that have successfully reduced burnout. Although every organization we described has not labeled their management approach as "Lean," they all share the philosophy and foundational principles of Lean Done Right. Working with physicians, organizational leaders can create work environments that foster physician well-being and achievement of the Triple Aim.

We begin with our recommendations for executive leaders, because our experience and interviews with experts have convinced us that their action is critical in addressing the workplace problems that drive physician burnout. Next, we list our recommendations for board members. These individuals play an important role in ensuring that the drivers of burnout are addressed because they have ultimate responsibility for the financial well-being of the organization, which burnout will adversely affect, because they can direct necessary resources toward addressing the underlying problems that drive burnout, and because they are responsible for hiring and ensuring the effectiveness of the CEO. Last, we present our recommendations for physicians. Physicians play a pivotal role in addressing burnout not only by seeking help personally if needed and by advocating for wellness programs but also by actively engaging with leaders in identifying and mitigating the underlying factors that are making clinical work simply unsustainable in many organizations.

## RECOMMENDATIONS FOR EXECUTIVE LEADERS

Executive leaders must take action in two primary ways. They must build the capacity of the organization to address burnout, and they must take targeted action to fix the underlying drivers of burnout on all three levels: individual physician, workplace drivers, and external drivers.

## BUILDING CAPACITY

Building the capacity of your organization to address burnout requires that you adopt processes for identifying the incidence of burnout and uncovering its causes and for building your knowledge about burnout.

**Learn about burnout at your organization.** It is absolutely essential that you gather information so that you and your leadership team are knowledgeable about burnout in general and about the incidence and impact of burnout at your organization in particular.

To gather information, we recommend the following three steps:

1. Conduct regular surveys of physicians to monitor the incidence of burnout, and identify sources of dissatisfaction. Consider using some of the surveys listed in the two sections that follow. *Burnout incidence*
   - Maslach Burnout Inventory (MBI): widely used burnout survey created by Christina Maslach and Michael Leiter; available for a fee at www.mindgarden.com.
   - Mini-Z Burnout Survey: short survey created by Mark Linzer; available free through the American Medical Association at www.stepsforward.org.
   *Sources of dissatisfaction*
   - Areas of Worklife Survey: companion to MBI; available for a fee at www.mindgarden.com; note that a version is available that also includes the MBI.
   - American Medical Group Association's physician satisfaction survey: survey created by AMGA; available for a fee through its Provider Satisfaction Benchmarking Program at www.amga.org.
2. Go to the *gemba* to see the existing barriers and frustrations. Create opportunities to speak with physicians to learn their concerns. Here are some strategies for creating these opportunities.
   - Spend time regularly in the physician lounge and the lunchroom.
   - Convene and meet regularly with a physician advisory council.
   - Schedule a regular dinner meeting with small groups of physicians from a variety of fields.

- When rounding in the clinical areas, ask physicians and staff to show you specific barriers or frustrations they are encountering.
- Regularly shadow physicians for a couple of hours at a time to see how they work and where they encounter barriers to their work.
- Consider creating a formalized mechanism for receiving feedback from frontline clinicians. (See the description of Mission Health System's WikiWisdom in Chapter 10.)

3. Build your knowledge of burnout. Use various resources to gain a better understanding of the problem.
   - Read articles about how other organizations are addressing burnout.
   - Subscribe to blog sites that focus on burnout.
   - Read books about burnout. (See Appendix 1 for a recommended reading list.)
   - Attend presentations, meetings, and workshops on burnout.
   - Join a site visit to an organization that is addressing burnout successfully.

**Take proactive steps to create a Lean culture founded in Respect for People.** Deep and sustained organizational change requires that you change how you lead, which in turn requires that you change where you spend your time, how you interact with others, and the messages you communicate to those you lead. Changing the way you lead requires that you undergo a personal transformation.

In our experience, leaders who value and respect their workforce in a highly personal way have undergone a profound personal transformation that results in greater humility, greater comfort with vulnerability, and acknowledgment of the limitations of their personal knowledge and ability.

To foster a culture of respect, we recommend the following steps:

1. Conduct an honest self-evaluation.
2. Learn about alternatives to Sloan-style, top-down management.

3. In executive meetings, use storytelling and modeling of respect and other desired behaviors to shift culture by demonstrating, "This is how we do things here."
4. Build your knowledge of Lean. Here are some specific action steps for learning more about Lean.
   - Read about Lean. (See Appendix 1 for a recommended reading list.)
   - Attend a conference on Lean in Health Care that includes a focus session on leadership.
   - Join a Lean study trip to see firsthand how Lean organizations perform.
   - Solicit help from a seasoned Lean coach, either inside your organization or through a consultancy.
   - Consider carefully the requirements for Lean leadership and the need for a personal transformation in your leadership approach.
   - Launch an A3 process (outlined in Appendix 2) focused on physician burnout to better understand the underlying drivers at your organization and to develop an action plan for addressing them.

## TAKING ACTION

After building the capacity of your organization to address physician burnout, it is essential that you implement strategies to address the three levels of burnout drivers.

**Identify prevention and treatment of burnout as a key strategic priority.** You can take several steps to prioritize addressing burnout. We recommend the following steps:

1. Include burnout as an agenda item for all executive meetings.
2. Add burnout and wellness metrics to your organizational performance dashboard.
3. Clearly communicate to any direct reports who are not fully engaged in tackling the issue that addressing physician burnout is a priority for you.

**Start a physician wellness program.** The program can address the individual physician factors that drive burnout and can help physicians with active burnout symptoms or other forms of distress.

We recommend these steps:

1. Empower physicians to lead the program.
2. Review and refine confidentiality policies to encourage use of the resources.
3. Provide adequate funding and other support.

**Implement a Lean management system.** A Lean management system (LMS) will allow you to identify and address the workplace drivers of burnout. As you adopt an LMS, we recommend that you adopt the following steps:

1. Make addressing burnout a key priority in your strategy deployment process.
2. Intensively redesign workflow, starting in one location. Choose the site based on weighted criteria, with burnout prevalence a significant factor in the weighting. After successfully redesigning the workflow at the pilot site, spread the redesign to other locations.
3. Implement the use of daily problem-solving huddles throughout your organization. Implement daily huddles first in patient care sites; later spread their use to non-clinical units. Implement tiered huddles to escalate problems quickly from front line to C-suite if needed. Train directors, managers, and supervisors to become effective coaches and mentors rather than problem-solving firefighters who mandate performance outcomes without providing support.
4. Use the Lean 5S process (a method for removing excess materials from the workplace and organizing required items) throughout your organization to reduce clutter and chaos in the workplace environment.
5. Identify and fix ubiquitous problems, such as the data-entry burden associated with the EHR. To do so, first create an optimization team to address a problem, reporting at the daily

huddles, with relevant information channeled to leadership through the tiered huddle process. Use Lean tools (for example, the A3 process) to identify underlying causes and develop an action plan.

**Bridge any existing gap between administration and physicians.** Success in addressing burnout requires that you involve physicians in developing a new organizational culture and in your strategic planning process. Some suggested steps include the following:

1. Work with physicians and other clinicians to define new vision, mission, and values (VMV) statements. Refer to the VMV statements when making both major and minor decisions. Start every meeting with a patient story, and draw the connection to the VMV statements.
2. Create a compact with physicians based on the new VMV statements.
3. Involve physicians in strategic planning.
4. Elicit input from frontline physicians. (See the descriptions in Chapter 10 of Mission Health System's WikiWisdom and Vancouver Clinic's use of a nominal group technique to involve physicians in strategic planning.)
5. Invite physician stakeholders from multiple specialties to work as a team to propose priorities in the capital budget.
6. Take steps to ensure that physicians are able to spend at least 10 to 20 percent of work time in the area that is most meaningful to them. Physicians often have a specific interest within their specialty or find working with a particular patient population to be especially meaningful.

   Ensuring time spent in an area of interest has been linked to lower burnout rates, as we discussed in Chapter 4, and is an effective way to demonstrate to physicians that you are listening to their values and are providing opportunities for change. Facilitate the pursuit of physicians' areas of interest and support physicians within a group in selecting different areas on which to focus. Building these areas of interest will not only reduce the risk of burnout but also may offer a competitive advantage to your organization—the differentiation of services may provide expertise that allows your organization to serve a broader patient population.

**Consider the impact of external pressures on physicians and take steps to minimize them.** Your efforts to affect policy at the local and national level can have an impact. We recommend the following steps when taking action to minimize the effects of external drivers:

1. Bring the physician perspective into your work with insurers or other external entities that develop regulations or legislation that affect health care delivery (for example, Centers for Medicare and Medicaid Services [CMS], Joint Commission, National Quality Forum [NQF]).
2. Advocate for changes in legislation and regulations to improve the physician experience.
3. Solicit input from physicians about the potential impact of new mandates and proactively take steps to mitigate their effect on physicians' daily practice.

## RECOMMENDATIONS FOR BOARD MEMBERS
(Note that many of these recommendations duplicate those we made for executive leaders.)

**Learn about burnout at your organization.** Gather information so that you and other members of the board are knowledgeable about burnout in general and about the incidence and impact of burnout at your organization in particular.

1. Go to the *gemba* to see the existing barriers and frustrations. (See the description of Mission Health System's Immersion Day in Chapter 10.) Talk to physicians to learn their concerns. Some strategies for creating opportunities to speak with physicians include the following:

- Visit them in the physician lounge or lunchroom.
- Hold a "Board Immersion Day" in which board members shadow physicians, nurses, and executives to see the work as it is being done.
- Speak with physician members of the board.
- Schedule a regular dinner meeting with physicians from a variety of fields.

2. Build your knowledge of burnout. Suggested steps include the following:
   - Read articles about how other organizations are addressing burnout.
   - Subscribe to blog sites that focus on burnout.
   - Read books about burnout. (See Appendix 1 for a recommended reading list.)
   - Attend presentations, meetings, and workshops on burnout.
   - Join executive leaders on a site visit to an organization that is addressing burnout successfully.

3. Build your knowledge of Lean.
   - Read about Lean. (See Appendix 1 for a recommended reading list.)
   - Join a Lean study trip to see firsthand how Lean organizations perform.
   - Solicit help from a seasoned Lean coach, either inside your organization or through a consultancy.

4. Evaluate whether your current CEO has the capacity for Lean leadership.

**Make burnout a priority.** As a board member, you hold the ultimate fiduciary responsibility for your organization. Physician burnout threatens the vitality and viability of health care organizations in several ways, with consequences and costs that we discussed in Chapter 2. We recommend the following steps to communicate that addressing burnout is a top priority:

1. Insist on a culture founded in Respect for People.
2. Include burnout as a board-meeting agenda item and give the topic as much attention as that given to quality and safety.

3. Communicate to your CEO the importance of addressing burnout. Consider building improvement in physician burnout scores into the metrics for the CEO's bonus, if appropriate.
4. Hold the CEO accountable for addressing burnout by supporting the distribution of needed resources for individual wellness programs and for fixing the workplace drivers of burnout. If the CEO is not addressing physician burnout and is not responding to your guidance regarding burnout, you need a new CEO. It is within the purview of the board to hire, guide, and, if necessary, fire the CEO.

**Take steps to minimize the external drivers of burnout.** Your efforts to affect policy at the local and national level can have an impact. We recommend the following steps when taking action to minimize the effects of external drivers:

1. Bring the physician perspective into your work with insurers or other external entities (for example, the CMS, Joint Commission, or NQF) that develop regulations or legislation that affects health care delivery.
2. Advocate for changes in legislation and regulations to improve the physician work experience.
3. Solicit input from physicians about the potential impact of new mandates and proactively take steps to mitigate the effects of these mandates on physicians' daily practice.

## RECOMMENDATIONS FOR PHYSICIANS

We have two overarching recommendations for physicians: take steps to address burnout in your own life, and seek out opportunities to lead. Being an active leader in your organization, whether informally or in a formal position, is the most effective way to impact the underlying drivers of burnout.

**Take steps to address your burnout symptoms.** If you are currently suffering from burnout, know that you are not alone, that burnout is neither your fault nor a sign of weakness, and that help is available.

Here are some steps to consider:

1. Reach out to others, seek professional help, step up self-care practices, and request time off if you need it.
2. If you're concerned about a colleague, speak directly to him or her about your concern.
3. Advocate for a physician burnout task force and wellness program at your organization.
4. Learn more about the risk factors and warning signs of physician suicide. (For more information, see the American Medical Association's Steps Forward modules on resiliency, burnout, and physician suicide at www.stepsforward.org.)

**Build your knowledge of burnout and of Lean.** Gaining knowledge about burnout and about Lean will help you better understand the drivers of physician burnout and potential strategies for change. Our recommendations include the following:

1. Read books or listen to audio books about burnout and Lean. (See Appendix 1 for a recommended reading list.)
2. Subscribe to blogs and podcasts that focus on Lean and burnout.
3. Read articles about the steps other organizations have taken to address burnout and to fix the workplace drivers of burnout.
4. Attend presentations, meetings, and workshops on burnout and Lean.
5. Join executive leaders on a site visit to an organization that is addressing burnout successfully.
6. Once your organization starts a Lean transformation, participate fully.
   - If asked, join or, better yet, lead a value stream steering team.
   - Participate in a rapid improvement event, even if it takes a week of your time.
   - Join in the daily huddles at your clinical site, helping your team identify and solve problems.

**Participate in improvement work to identify and remove the workplace drivers of burnout.** Don't get caught in an "eddy," believing that your situation cannot improve or that you are too busy to participate in redesigning the way the work is done. Inefficacy is a symptom of burnout; it's important to take concrete action steps to avoid being a victim of the lack of efficiency and forethought in the design of the health care system.

Think carefully about your priorities. Will you be better off next month or next year if you spend an hour, a day, or a week seeing patients in a chaotic work environment or if you dedicate that time to fixing the chaos? It's tempting to leave the work to someone else, but if you have read this book through to this point, you know a lot more than most about the issue and can be a valuable resource to your colleagues and your organization.

We recommend these two steps:

1. Seek out opportunities to develop your leadership skills.
2. Step into either a formal or an informal leadership role.

**Take an active role in improving your relationship with administration.** Bridging the gap between physicians and administration can seem like a loathsome task to many physicians, given the current state of affairs in many organizations today. Physicians can help executives understand the enormity of the impact of burnout, identify its origin in systems problems that also affect performance metrics, and recognize that cost-effective strategies exist to prevent it.

Our recommended steps include the following:

1. Approach your organizational leader as an individual, or preferably as a group, to voice your concerns about burnout. Suggest that they champion an A3 process as outlined in Appendix 2. If they are amenable to the A3, request a way to remain involved or, at a minimum, to be informed about the leadership team's progress.
2. If your leaders do not recognize the seriousness of the problem, gather and present data about the downstream effects of burnout on physicians, patients, and health care organizations. If they seem to be focused on finances, remind them that replacing a physician lost to early retirement, leaving practice, or suicide

is an expensive proposition—estimated to be at least $400,000 according to leaders we interviewed—and that reduced work schedules decrease the $1,400,000 a typical primary care doctor contributes to a hospital's revenue. (Merritt Hawkins 2016)

3. Request that they engage a burnout expert to present at Grand Rounds, with the goal of increasing physicians' and leaders' knowledge about burnout.

4. If you are unable to garner their attention sufficiently, run an A3 yourself. Approach your physician leader or gather a group of interested colleagues. If you are unable to obtain external expertise, look for a colleague with experience in Lean to lead the A3 within your practice, department, or unit.

5. If your leaders fail to acknowledge the seriousness of physician burnout at your organization, consider "voting with your feet." The stakes are too high to remain in a practice setting that increases your risk of experiencing the devastating consequences of burnout—medical errors, chronic dissatisfaction with your career, depression, and suicide.

**If you are doing well, consider taking the opportunity to help fellow physicians as a leader or mentor.** If you are drawn to leadership, take on a formal or informal leadership role. More physicians in the C-suite would be ideal. Physician executives can help non-physician leaders understand the challenges of the medical staff and help physicians understand the challenges that administrators face. Consider accessing opportunities for leadership training.

If you have found individual or workplace strategies that have helped you avoid or manage burnout, consider becoming a resource to your colleagues and sharing what has worked for you to help those who are struggling.

**To minimize the effects of the external drivers of burnout, take steps to influence health care policy.** Physicians' time for advocacy work is limited. However, as highly educated professionals, their voices make an impact. We suggest these steps:

1. Keep informed about potential policy changes and their implications for your practice and patient care.
2. Work with your state medical society and national specialty societies and professional groups to bring the physician perspective to the governmental agencies, insurers, and other external entities (for example, CMS, Joint Commission, or NQF) that develop regulations or legislation that affects health care delivery.

# CONCLUSION

Burnout has become an overwhelming problem—overwhelming for those individuals experiencing it, most definitely, and for leaders of health care organizations who are attempting to guide their hospitals and practices through the incredibly challenging climate that is health care today. Burnout adversely affects every stakeholder in the health care system. We cannot delay in addressing it.

If you are a physician, you have likely been personally affected by burnout, either your own or that of your colleagues. Take time to learn about the symptoms of burnout and how to identify the underlying drivers in your workplace. Work with administration to fix the root problems that are causing burnout and ultimately affecting your patients.

If you are a health care leader, you play an instrumental role in addressing the drivers of burnout. You must make a choice: will you be a part of the problem or a part of the solution?

Due to the severity and urgency of the problem, it is tempting to take the traditional approach of appointing a committee tasked with identifying and implementing best practices for burnout. In Chapter 10, we described the work of a number of organizations that could be considered best practices. You could simply try to implement those and would likely see some partial or temporary success.

You are also likely to find that what worked somewhere else can't be effectively "cut and pasted" into your organization. Every organization is different. Respecting what is unique about your organization and your physicians by taking a Lean approach and partnering with your physicians to support and empower them in solving the root causes of burnout in your organization will dramatically improve your chances of success.

Take the lead in transforming your organization through Lean Done Right, which is based in the principle of Respect for People. Lean Done Right will empower your physicians, prevent burnout, and give your organization an operational effectiveness and adaptability that may well be its greatest competitive advantage.

We strongly encourage you to take the steps laid out in this book, and lead a change for the better in your organization. For the sake of physicians, other clinicians, health care organizations, and patients, the time to act is now.

## REFERENCES

Merritt Hawkins. Physician inpatient/outpatient revenue survey. 2016. Available at: https://www.merritthawkins.com/uploadedFiles/MerrittHawkins/Surveys/Merritt_Hawkins-2016_RevSurvey.pdf. Accessed September 27, 2016.

# Appendix 1: Recommended Reading List

## BURNOUT
### Books
Leiter MP, Bakker AB, Maslach C, eds. *Burnout at Work: A Psychological Perspective.* New York: Psychological Press. 2014.

Maslach C, Leiter M. *The Truth About Burnout: How Organizations Cause Personal Stress and What to Do About It.* San Francisco: Jossey-Bass. 2000.

Murphy T. *Physician Burnout: A Guide to Recognition and Recovery.* Aloha Publishing. 2015.

### Articles
Bodenheimer T, Sinsky C. From triple to quadruple aim: care of the patient requires care of the provider. *Ann Fam Med.* 2014;12(6):573–576.

Linzer M, Manwell LB, Williams ES, et al.; MEMO (Minimizing Error, Maximizing Outcome) Investigators. Working conditions in primary care: physician reactions and care quality. *Ann Intern Med.* 2009;151(1):28–36.

Maslach C, Leiter MP. Early predictors of job burnout and engagement. *J Appl Psychol.* 2008;93(3):498–512.

Shanafelt TD, Gorringe G, Menaker R, et al. Impact of organizational leadership on physician burnout and satisfaction. *Mayo Clin Proc.* 2015;90(4):432–440.

Shanafelt TD, Hasan O, Dyrbye LN, et al. Changes in burnout and satisfaction with work-life balance in physicians and the general US working population between 2011 and 2014. *Mayo Clin Proc.* 2015;90(12):1600–1613.

Shanafelt TD, Mungo M, Schmitgen J, et al. Longitudinal study evaluating the association between physician burnout and changes in professional work effort. *Mayo Clin Proc.* 2016;91(4):422–431.

Sinsky CA, Willard-Grace R, Schutzbank AM, Sinsky TA, Margolius D, Bodenheimer T. In search of joy in practice: a report of 23 high-functioning primary care practices. *Ann Fam Med.* 2013;11(3):272–278.

*Other Media*

Bromley E. Pediatric ground rounds: physician burnout, depression, and demoralization. [Presentation]. 2014. Available at: http://www.uctv.tv/shows/28597.

American Medical Association. Steps Forward. [Online modules on preventing physician burnout and other topics related to practice improvement]. Available at: www.stepsforward.org.

## LEADERSHIP

Chapman B, Sisodia R. *Everybody Matters: The Extraordinary Power of Caring for Your People Like Family.* New York: Penguin Random House. 2015.

Pink DH. *Drive: The Surprising Truth About What Motivates Us.* New York: Riverhead Books. 2011.

Sinek S. *Leaders Eat Last: Why Some Teams Pull Together and Others Don't.* New York: Penguin Group. 2014.

## LEAN

Albanese C, Aaby D, Platchek TS. *Advanced Lean in Healthcare.* North Charleston, SC: CreateSpace. 2014

Barnas K, Adams E. *Beyond Heroes: A Lean Management System for Healthcare.* Appleton, WI: The ThedaCare Center for Healthcare Value. 2014.

Cooper C. *The Little Book of Lean: The Basics.* Bloomfield, IN: Simpler Consulting. 2011.

Gabow PA, Goodman PL. *The Lean Prescription: Powerful Medicine for Our Ailing Healthcare System.* Boca Raton, FL: Productivity Press. 2015.

Graban M. *Lean Hospitals: Improving Quality, Patient Safety, and Employee Engagement, 3rd edition.* Boca Raton, FL: CRC Press. 2016.

Hafer MS. *Simpler Healthcare: Using Lean to Achieve Breakthrough Improvements in Safety, Quality, Access, and Productivity.* Charleston, SC: Simpler Healthcare. 2012.

Institute for Healthcare Improvement. *Going Lean in Health Care.* IHI Innovation Series white paper. Cambridge, MA: Institute for Healthcare Improvement. 2005.

Koenigsaecker G. *Leading the Lean Enterprise Transformation.* Boca Raton, FL: CRC Press. 2013.

Toussaint J, Adams E. *Management on the Mend: The Healthcare Executive Guide to System Transformation.* Appleton, WI: The ThedaCare Center for Healthcare Value. 2015.

Toussaint J, Gerard RA, Adams E. *On the Mend: Revolutionizing Healthcare to Save Lives and Transform the Industry.* Cambridge, MA: Lean Enterprise Institute Inc. 2010.

Wellman J, Hagan P, Jeffries H. *Leading the Lean Healthcare Journey: Driving Culture Change to Increase Value.* New York: Productivity Press. 2011.

# Appendix 2: Illustration of A3 Process

Although there are many A3 formats available, we prefer a nine-box A3 because it is well suited for organizations that are new to Lean; it clearly walks through the steps in the A3 process. As shown in figure 4, each box in the A3 document represents a step in the process. The rest of this section describes how to work through an A3 on physician burnout for a hypothetical health care organization, which we'll call ABC Health System.

We describe the process with the assumption that senior leaders are engaged and supportive, although leaders or supervisors at any level can initiate an A3. Please note that applying the specific findings in this example to your organization would threaten the success of the endeavor—the strength of the A3 activity lies in the fact-finding, team-building process itself. The A3 process, done right, is iterative and best completed with a great deal of discussion and refinement and with multiple iterations over time.

In this scenario, the ABC leaders have decided to use an A3 to address physician burnout at their large, academic, integrated health system. They have decided to focus first on physicians in inpatient settings at the flagship hospital.

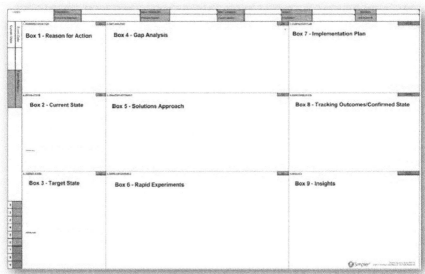

Figure 4: Example of A3 Document

## TOP AND SIDE BOXES: IDENTIFYING THE PROJECT AND TEAM MEMBERS

In the title box, the ABC leadership team specifies the name of the project—in this case, "Preventing physician burnout at ABC Health System." They identify the CEO as the executive sponsor, responsible for ensuring that the initiative receives needed prioritization and resources, and the CMO as the value stream owner, responsible for managing the process over its course.

In the site/location box, the team specifies "inpatient units of the flagship hospital," because they want to focus on understanding and addressing the burnout drivers that are most important for each particular site. In the team members' box, they list key people by title who will be actively engaged in the A3. They identify 10 people: several C-suite members—the CMO, the CMIO, and the CFO—two members of the board, and five physician leaders representing various service lines.

## BOX 1: REASON FOR ACTION

In the reason for action box, the ABC leaders list the problem statement. They write, "We recognize that physician burnout is a significant problem across the country and within our organization, impacting many of our physicians. We recognize that burnout is adversely affecting physicians personally and causing negative effects on quality, safety, and the patient experience. To achieve the Triple Aim, the problem needs to be corrected. We are committed to fixing the problem for the benefit of everyone in our organization. Although we recognize that burnout affects other professionals in our organization, we are focusing on physician burnout in this A3."

## BOX 2: INITIAL STATE

In this box, the leadership team describes the initial state. To do so, they first identify the quantitative and qualitative metrics they will monitor to assess improvement in physician burnout. They decide to use the Maslach Burnout Inventory (MBI), scoring all three symptom dimensions (emotional exhaustion, depersonalization, and inefficacy) to determine the prevalence of burnout. They also select several parameters from the AGMA physician satisfaction survey to better understand the drivers of burnout at their organization and within specific departments. Finally, for balance, they select several other metrics related to quality, safety, and patient experience to ensure that other aspects of performance are not negatively impacted by interventions to prevent burnout.

The leaders depict the initial state qualitatively by creating a drawing of an ED physician pounding in frustration at the computer keyboard in the midst of a chaotic environment with patients lined up on gurneys awaiting admission while a full waiting room of patients frowns and yells in anger about delays. Although the drawing process seems frivolous given the seriousness of the problem, the team finds the experience helpful and engaging.

## BOX 3: TARGET STATE

In Box 3, the team clarifies their goal with quantitative targets ensuring that the goals were challenging and will result in meaningful reduction in burnout while also being achievable for a first pass at addressing the problem. As a basic tenet, Lean coaches often suggest "halving the bad and doubling the good." The leaders select a balanced set of targets. They decide, for example, to set the goal of moving from the 35th percentile for physician satisfaction to the 55th percentile.

To describe the target state qualitatively, they draw a companion piece to the initial state drawing. In this depiction, the physician is smiling and waiting to see the next patient, with a nearly empty waiting room and a transport technician wheeling away the only patient awaiting admission.

## BOX 4: GAP ANALYSIS

The leaders then conduct a gap analysis. They search for explanations for the gaps between the initial state and the target state. This process involves identifying the underlying causes of burnout for physicians at the flagship hospital. To do this, they go to the clinical care areas to talk with and observe the frontline physicians in the hospital. They identify many inefficiencies, delays, errors, and frustrations that the physicians are encountering.

Once they identify these gaps, they list these on the "fishbone diagram" in Box 4 that groups the gaps into categories with similar attributes. Using a Pareto analysis, the ABC leaders identify five major gaps: lack of communication between administration and physicians, issues with EHR usability, excessive time burden associated with documentation, delays in getting consults completed, and lack of coordination between central scheduling and the inpatient units.

They then dig deep into the root causes of these gaps using a common Lean tool, the Five Whys. For example, for the first identified gap, these are their questions and responses.

1. Why is there a lack of communication between administration and physicians? Because administrators are busy in meetings all day.
2. Why are administrators in meetings all day? Because they are trying to improve the hospital's performance on the 30 quality metrics on their balanced scorecard.
3. Why are they trying to improve the performance on the quality metrics? Because the hospital needs the increased revenues that are tied to better performance on quality metrics.
4. Why does the hospital need the increased revenues? To fund physician recruiting because they have high physician turnover.
5. Why do they have high physician turnover? Because the physicians' needs are not being addressed.

The Five Whys approach will also be used for other key gaps to identify a representative set of root causes.

## BOX 5: SOLUTIONS APPROACH

The solutions approach in Box 5 uses an "if we, then we" logic to consider one or more actions that would address the identified root causes. For example, to address the root cause of the physicians' needs not being met, one solution would be, "If we create a physician council that meets regularly with senior leaders, then the CEO and other leaders will better understand physicians' needs."

## BOX 6: RAPID EXPERIMENTS

Box 6 lists the rapid experiments the team will conduct to see if the potential solutions listed in Box 5 are effective. To test the effectiveness of forming a physicians' council, the group decides to develop the council, hold monthly meetings, and survey physician members of the council one week after each meeting to ensure the physicians' needs were being heard and addressed.

## BOX 7: COMPLETION PLAN

In Box 7, the leaders describe the plan for completing the initiative, specifying what, who, and when for each action step. They list specific actions, owners, the due dates, and the actual completion date. They use a color code for each action: green if the action was on track and red if it was not. For example, ABC leaders list "formalize the physician council" as an action, list the CMO as the owner, and identify a due date.

## BOX 8: CONFIRMED STATE

In Box 8, the leaders track the metrics identified in Boxes 2 and 3. They assess the monthly and quarterly results to see whether they were on target for achieving their year-end goals.

For example, they find that an internal survey conducted regularly and validated by annual MBI and AMGA provider satisfaction surveys shows improvement in the metrics they are tracking. If some metrics are not improving, the A3 team will focus on those metrics and develop countermeasures to get them back on track.

## BOX 9: INSIGHTS

In Box 9, the team lists lessons learned that would help form the basis for future A3s, including the one they planned to conduct next: addressing burnout among primary care physicians in the health system's seven community-based clinics and eight group practices.

# INDEX

# More About the Authors

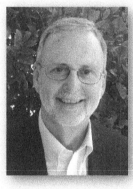

Dr. Paul DeChant practiced family medicine for 25 years and has 30 years of health care management experience, including as a medical director, department chair, CEO, and board member. He now serves as an executive coach and senior advisor with Simpler(r) Healthcare. Having experienced the power of leading Lean transformations, Paul is passionate about improving the lives of clinicians, staff, patients, and leaders in health care organizations - and helping physicians thrive in a collaborative and supportive work environment. You can find Paul on the web at pauldechantmd.com and on Twitter @pauldechantmd.

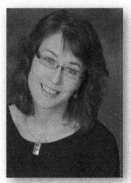

Dr. Diane Shannon is a freelance writer, physician advocate, and change agent. She's also an internist who left medical practice due to burnout. Diane writes on topics such as the patient experience, communication, patient safety, communication, electronic health records, and teamwork. Diane first wrote publicly about her experience with burnout in 2013 in a post for WBUR, the Boston National Public Radio affiliate. The many physicians who share their personal stories of burnout are the motivation for this book and for her work. You can find Diane on the web at mdwriter.com and on Twitter @dianewshannon.

CPSIA information can be obtained
at www.ICGtesting.com
Printed in the USA
LVHW02s2339060318
568948LV00006B/225/P